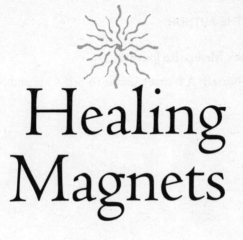

Healing Magnets

The Nurse's Meditative Journal

Healing Yourself: A Nurse's Guide to Self-Care and Renewal

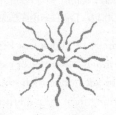

Healing Magnets

A guide for pain relief,
speeding recovery,
and restoring balance

Sherry Kahn, M.P.H.

THREE RIVERS PRESS • NEW YORK

Published by Three Rivers Press, New York, New York. Member of the Crown Publishing Group.

Random House, Inc. New York, Toronto, London, Sydney, Auckland

www.randomhouse.com

Three Rivers Press is a registered trademark and the Three Rivers Press colophon is a trademark of Random House, Inc.

Printed in the United States of America

Designed by Susan Maksuta

Library of Congress Cataloging-in-Publication Data
Kahn, Sherry.
    Healing magnets : a guide for pain relief, speeding recovery, and
restoring balance / by Sherry Kahn.
       p.   cm.
    Includes bibliographical references and index.
    I. Magnetotherapy.   I. Title.
  RM893.K346   2000
  615.8'45—dc21   99-058303

ISBN 0–609–80555–X

10   9   8   7   6   5   4   3   2   1

First Edition

IMPORTANT NOTICE

This book provides exciting information about magnet therapy, from which many people have benefited. You should, however, see a physician if you have acute or persistent undiagnosed pain. Such pain may indicate a serious problem that may require more sophisticated intervention than magnet therapy.

The author has no financial interest in any manufacturer or distributor of therapeutic magnets.

CONTENTS

ACKNOWLEDGMENTS

It may take a village to raise a child—but let me tell you, it also takes a village to write a book like this!

First of all, I thank all the magnet therapy practitioners, researchers, and distributors who consented to interviews. Next, I thank all the people who assisted me by providing information, resources, and manuscript feedback, including Lorri Beaver, D.C.; Lela Carney, L.Ac.; Serafina Corsello, M.D.; Gloria Garland; Ron Galbavy; Daytra Hansel; Mary Hardy, M.D.; Hamsa Henry, L.Ac., O.M.D.; Anna Katarina; Dan Lobash, Ph.D., L.Ac.; Tom Nellesen; Mileva Saulo, Ed.D., R.N.; Stephen Stiteler, L.Ac., O.M.D.; Kathy Wanderer, R.N.; and Carl Wirz. Special thanks for technical clarification goes to John Zimmerman, Ph.D. I also thank artist Gail Hada-Insley for the appendix 2 drawings.

On the literary side, I am grateful to my agent, Sarah Jane Freymann, for her continuing support and for allowing me to graduate from the Freymann School for Wayward Writers, and to Three Rivers Press and editors Teryn Johnson, Jessica Schulte, and Kristen Wolfe for bringing this information to the public.

FOREWORD

More and more Americans are getting interested in using magnets for self-healing. And finally, there is a book on magnet therapy that I can recommend without reservation to both my patients and colleagues.

As a physician who uses primarily natural healing modalities, I'm always on the lookout for nontoxic, noninvasive healing tools. I first discovered magnets more than a decade ago. I have personally found them useful and include them among the energy medicine tools we use in my centers. But I have been frustrated, as have many others, by the lack of clear, unbiased information on the subject of magnet therapy.

Sherry Kahn, with her propensity for digging deep and her talent for transforming technical material into accessible, entertaining prose, brings a much-needed clarity to this confusing topic. You will find the chapters on how to choose and use magnets for self-care particularly useful. Here, at last, are pragmatic guidelines for sorting through the many available magnetic products so that you can make wise purchasing decisions. With a variety of options for using magnets clearly laid out, you can get started without hesitation.

For those who relish the latest expert thinking on the subject, as I do, this book provides a summary of the theories and an international overview of research on the many conditions that respond to magnet therapy. A good deal of this information—not available through conventional sources—is being made available to the public for the first time.

Healing Magnets separates fiction from fact. In digestible bites, it explains the science behind the practice. It tells us what we know about magnet therapy and what we're still learning. With this book as a guide, anyone can safely and effectively use magnets to relieve pain, speed recovery, and balance energy.

SERAFINA CORSELLO, M.D., F.A.C.A.M.
CORSELLO CENTERS FOR INTEGRATIVE MEDICINE
NEW YORK, NEW YORK

Healing Magnets

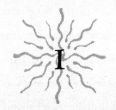

An Ancient Tool
for Modern Times

Legend has it that Cleopatra wore a magnet on her forehead because she believed it would keep her young and beautiful. Ancient texts from India and China speak of the healing powers of magnetic stones. The Greeks called them "live stones" (*lapis vivus* in Latin) because they seemed to have lives of their own—inexplicably moving toward each other and any object containing iron. For thousands of years, we humans have been fascinated by magnets. Each century, we learn a little bit more about how and why they work as healing tools.

Today, our scientists are providing us with evidence that supports the experiences of the earliest users of healing magnets. In the new millennium—a time of increasing openness to natural remedies and energy medicine—magnet therapy is rapidly gaining popularity as a treatment for many modern-day maladies. Why? First of all, it works. Anecdotal healing reports abound.

A pain relief success rate in the 80 percent range is a common finding among both clinicians and researchers. It is safe. And magnets are inexpensive and easy to use on your own. Cathy's experience is like the stories of so many other people, including well-known athletes, who have tried magnet therapy.

CATHY'S STORY

Cathy is a self-employed word processor. At times, she can spend as much as fourteen hours a day at her computer. After an uninterrupted four months of such a demanding schedule, Cathy found that her "mouse hand" was sore. It had also become weak. Everyday activities that she had previously never thought about, such as picking up a gallon bottle of water, became painful experiences.

As Cathy prefers natural approaches for healing her ailments, she sought out the counsel of a chiropractor, who performed a variety of diagnostic tests. The good news was that it wasn't carpal tunnel syndrome. The bad news was that it was tendinitis—a painful inflammation of the tendons. The doctor adjusted her wrist and recommended anti-inflammatory herbs. Cathy returned to her chiropractor for several more adjustments and faithfully took her herbs. Although the wrist began to feel a little better, it was far from healed and continued to be aggravated by Cathy's unrelenting work schedule.

A friend who had recently injured his knee playing basketball with some younger friends told Cathy how he had applied a magnet to his knee and it had healed in a fraction of the time expected by his physician. Cathy ordered a magnetic wrap and applied it to her wrist. By the end of the week, she noticed that her wrist was both stronger and less painful. A month later, she was typing pain-free and was able to comfortably lift objects that previously had been troublesome.

MAGNETIC VERSUS ELECTROMAGNETIC FIELDS

Often, people use the terms *electromagnetic fields* and *magnetic fields* interchangeably. They are actually quite different and have different effects on our bodies. Electromagnetic fields are constantly moving and generating both electric and magnetic energies. When your computer is plugged in but not turned on, it emanates an electric field because there is voltage in the wire. However, when your computer is turned on and an electrical current moves through the wire, an electromagnetic field is generated. Exposure to extremely low frequency (ELF) electromagnetic fields, such as those generated by our everyday appliances and office equipment, has been linked with a wide array of health problems, including birth defects, reproductive dysfunction, cancer, and neurological disorders. Scientists have recently documented that ELF electromagnetic fields adversely impact the thyroid, thymus, and pineal—endocrine glands essential for normal metabolic functioning.[1]

Static magnets, which are the ones people are using for self-healing, are stationary and emanate only magnetic fields. Unlike electromagnetic fields, static magnetic fields have been found to be completely safe, even at the tremendous strengths of magnetic resonance imaging (MRI) machines, commonly used for medical diagnosis.

A HELPFUL THERAPY FOR MANY AILMENTS

Today, the use of magnets for healing is an accepted medical therapy in Japan, China, Korea, Switzerland, Germany, and many Eastern European countries (including the former Soviet Union). Over the last few decades, researchers have reported on the beneficial effects of magnet therapy for both chronic and acute conditions, and I note many of those specific findings in later chapters. Currently, static magnets are used most frequently for the relief of pain from such conditions as arthritis, rheumatism, tendinitis and bursitis, back problems, headaches, muscle strains and sprains, carpal tunnel syndrome, and fibromyalgia. Static magnets have also been found to be helpful in accelerating the healing of injuries and wounds. Researchers have reported, for example, that the application of magnets speeds postsurgery recovery time.

Magnetic blankets have been used for many years to enhance the performance of racehorses. Many athletes—such as pro golfer Jim Colbert, baseball pitcher Hideki Irabu, and football linebacker Bill Romanowski—are devoted magnet users. They credit the magnets with both enhancing their performance and increasing their endurance.[2]

MAGNETIC FIELDS AND HEALTH

Pioneering orthopedic surgeon, researcher, and Nobel Prize nominee Dr. Robert O. Becker was one of the first to prove that our bodies are electromagnetic entities and that they are responsive to magnetic fields. In his fascinating book *The Body Electric: Electromagnetism and the Foundation of Life,*[3] Becker describes his study of psychiatric patients in the late 1950s. He and a colleague matched the admissions of more than twenty-eight thousand patients at eight hospitals against sixty-seven magnetic storms during a four-year period. They discovered that significantly more people were admitted just after magnetic storms than when the magnetic field was stable. Later research conducted by Becker confirmed these original findings and went on to prove that abnormal magnetic fields produce a wide range of physiological and psychological abnormalities in humans.

We learned more about the interaction of magnetic fields with our bodies from the first astronauts. The sickness they exhibited upon returning home was discovered to have been caused by the lack of magnetic fields in outer space. Space program researchers, in fact, found that mice raised in cages shielded from the earth's field lost their fur and began to die within a few weeks after being placed in such an environment.[4] In subsequent flights, NASA placed magnets in both the spaceships and the astronauts' space suits.

Scientists who have been able to measure the earth's magnetic field have noted that its strength has decreased about tenfold over the last 4,000 years.[5] Researchers such as Dr. Kyoichi Nakagawa believe that this decrease in the earth's field has resulted in magnetic field deficiency syndrome—characterized by symptoms such as fatigue, insomnia, frequent headaches, and generalized aches and pains.[6] Many believe that static magnets can restore the body's magnetic field. Once that field is in a state of natural balance, deficiency symptoms simply disappear.

Cleopatra may really have been on to something. That magnet she wore on her forehead to keep her young and beautiful was in line with the pineal gland, located in the center of the brain. The pineal gland, we now know, secretes melatonin—a hormone that researchers are discovering has many antiaging properties. Magnet therapists such as Swiss naturopath Holger Hannemann recommend the application of magnets to specific points on the face to tone muscles and improve skin circulation.[7] Some American companies even sell masks with attached magnets, specifically designed for such a nonsurgical face-lift.

WHO CAN USE MAGNETS

The beauty of magnets is that just about anyone can use them for self-care. There are only a few situations in which magnets should not be used. These precautions are addressed in chapter 7.

Magnet therapy is being practiced by a growing number of health-care professionals, including physicians, naturopaths, acupuncturists, chiropractors, and massage therapists. In fact, formal training programs in the art and science of magnet therapy, developed by leading experts, are beginning to be offered.

Magnet therapy is natural, safe, inexpensive, and easy to do. In the pages that follow, you will learn more about the science behind the practice and the pragmatics of how to use magnets to help yourself and your loved ones.

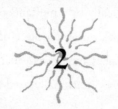

The History of Magnet Therapy

BACK TO THE BEGINNING

Magnet therapy is both an ancient practice and a frontier science. What is now being investigated by our scientists and physicians was first put into practice at least four thousand years ago.

Historical records track the use of magnets for healing our bodies' ills back to around 2000 B.C. It was then that the oldest known medical treatise, *The Yellow Emperor's Book of Internal Medicine,* was penned. In what would become the bible of traditional Chinese medicine, Houang-Ti laid out approaches to treating internal body imbalances by introducing external energy.

One such way of doing so was the insertion of needles in energetically charged points—a practice we know as acupuncture. Another therapeutic way of influencing these points and their associated energy channels (meridians) was through the application of lodestones. One ancient text describes how to treat deafness magnetically by simultaneously placing a mixture of herbs in the patient's ear and a piece of iron in the patient's mouth. A contemporary Chinese veterinary medicine text indicates that magnets were traditionally used to treat horses as well as people.[1]

It is believed that the Vedas, the religious scriptures of the Hindus, came into being around the same time as the Yellow Emperor's treatise. The Vedas' extensive teachings included descriptions of treatments for a wide variety of ailments using *ashmana* or *siktavati*—instruments of stone that many suspect were lodestones.

Interestingly, both traditional Chinese and Indian medicine (Ayurveda) are based on the concept of health's being dependent on the unimpeded flow of life force. The Chinese call it *chi* or *qi*, while the Indians call it *prana*. Both systems also speak of channels connected with energy distribution. In Chinese medicine, these are the meridians, while the Indian esoteric literature speaks of *nadis*.

The ancient Egyptians viewed all forms of illness as imbalances between the patient and the cosmos. Like the Chinese and Indians, the Egyptians believed that physical disease was a result of energetic imbalances. Gemstones were a very important part of their culture, and many believe that knowledge of the unique healing properties of these various minerals and crystals originated with the Egyptian healer priests. As noted in chapter I, it is widely claimed that Cleopatra wore a lodestone on her fore-head to maintain her youthfulness and beauty. Temple and tomb paintings are replete with images of Egyptians communicating and healing (electromagnetically) through their hands.

When we look at the seventh century B.C., we find Thales of Miletus, a Greek mathematician and philosopher who preceded Hippocrates (the Father of Medicine) by a couple of hundred years, connecting lodestones with some type of animated spirit. Some feel that Hippocrates's fifth-century B.C. writings indicate that he used magnets to assist the body in its self-healing process.[2] And Aristotle is reputed to have spoken of the thera-peutic properties of magnets.[3]

MOVING FORWARD

The next major landmark along the magnet therapy pathway is the sixteenth-century Swiss physician, chemist, and mystic Paracelsus. Paracelsus's studies took him across Europe and to the corners of Asia. Although he studied at many universities, he sought out "old wives, gypsies, sorcerers, wandering tribes, old robbers and such outlaws" as teachers.[4] Paracelsus challenged many of the conventional medical ideas of the time—one of the predominant ones being that there was a single cause and cure for every disease. He believed, like Hippocrates, that the body can heal itself, and his understanding of "like cures like" provided the basis for the later development of homeopathy.

Paracelsus believed, as the ancient Egyptians did, in a life force that was connected to the cosmos. He used natural forces to heal the body, including lodestone. He believed the body's life force, which he called *archaeus,* could be influenced by magnets. In fact, he believed magnets were more effective in curing many diseases and inflammations than any other natural remedy, and he used them to treat a wide variety of maladies. Paracelsus proclaimed, "The magnet is the king of all secrets." Five centuries later, we are still unraveling its mysteries, secret by secret.

In England, William Gilbert, physician to Queen Elizabeth I, not only proved that the earth was a large magnet but in his book *De Magnete,* published in 1600, defined magnetism and electricity as related but separate forces. He used lodestone in treating many diseases.

Franz Anton Mesmer is perhaps the most colorful figure in the history of magnet therapy. Mesmer was trained in medicine, mathematics, and law. His thinking was influenced by the ideas of Paracelsus and Maximillian Hell, an astronomer and Jesuit priest, who treated patients with steel magnets, made into the shape of the body organs to which they were applied.

Like Paracelsus, Mesmer believed in a cosmic life force. This universal force or fluid, he believed, was concentrated in animal nervous systems and magnets. He coined the term *animal magnetism* in 1766 to describe this force in living organisms, which he distinguished from the force concentrated in magnets, *mineral magnetism.* Based on his observation that the course of diseases fluctuated in response to the movement of the planets and other heavenly bodies, Mesmer concluded that the body fluids possessed polarities that could be influenced by external magnetic forces.

Mesmer's work included the treatment of disease both with magnets and with the animal magnetic force emitted from his hands—what we would today call "energy healing" or "laying on of hands." In Paris, the flamboyant Mesmer created a dramatic healing salon, where patients sat in wooden tubs, which contained both magnetized water and iron rods called *bacquets.* The setting was quite theatrical, complete with music, colored lights, and fabrics. Patients would hold on to the rods, and sometimes each other, to facilitate the flow of the universal fluid—with Mesmer adding to the force with either his hands or another magnetized rod.

Although Mesmer was discredited by the medical authorities of the time, and we find the term *mesmerism* to this day defined in our dictionaries as "hypnotism," modern experiments provide evidence that he really was onto something. In the 1970s, chemist Dr. Robert Miller found that when water was exposed both to magnets and to magnetic energy emitted from the hands of energy healers, the surface tension of the water was reduced. Furthermore, Miller discovered that when metal stirring rods were placed in contact with this altered water, the healing energy flowed in a specific direction—exactly what Mesmer claimed was happening in his salon healings.

In a later experiment, Miller watered seedlings with three types of water—regular tap water, healer-treated water, and magnet-treated water. In contrast to the tap-watered seeds, which had an 8 percent germination rate, healer-treated seeds had a 36 percent germination rate, while the magnet-treated seeds showed a 68 percent rate.[5] This experiment confirmed another of Mesmer's ideas—the relationship between animal magnetism and mineral magnetism.

MAGNET THERAPY IN THE UNITED STATES

In the United States, magnet therapy came to the forefront when Connecticut physician Elisha Perkins was given a patent in 1795 for his magnetic tractor. This handheld little device was gently and repeatedly moved by the practitioner over the afflicted body part to "pull off" the energetic field that Perkins believed was the source of the malady.

The use of static magnets became very popular after the Civil War, with a variety of "cure-all" products being sold through mail-order catalogs. The advent of AC (alternating-current) power, a few decades later, gave inventors the tools to develop electromagnetic healing devices. Electromagnetic therapy, included in the medical textbooks of the day, became an accepted treatment for a while for a wide variety of ailments.

With unsubstantiated and exaggerated claims, and the advent of effective antibiotics and other "miracle drugs," magnet therapy fell by the wayside in this country. For several decades now, we have relied on pharmaceuticals to cure the bulk of our ailments.

But the "wonder drugs" are turning out not to be so wonderful. Every year, more than 1 million Americans are hospitalized because of adverse drug reactions.[6] Many of us have been so overmedicated with antibiotics that they frequently don't work anymore. Popular painkillers—nonsteroidal anti-inflammatory drugs (or NSAIDS), like aspirin and ibuprofen (Advil, Aleve, Motrin)—can cause gastrointestinal bleeding, ulcers, and kidney damage if they are used continuously.[7] And acetaminophen (Tylenol) can damage the liver.[8]

Now, as more and more of us are seeking natural alternatives to potentially toxic drugs, magnet therapy is undergoing a revival in this country. Today, we know a little more than our predecessors about how and why magnets heal, and researchers and clinicians around the world are busy unveiling more of their secrets every day.

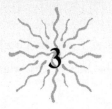

The Nature of Magnets

WHAT MAKES A MAGNET A MAGNET

Magnets are so much a part of our lives these days that we basically take them for granted. Small ones hold our grocery lists firmly on our refrigerator doors, while larger ones pull the doors shut. Without them, we couldn't watch television or read the contents of floppy disks on our computer monitors. The magnetic strips on the backs of credit and debit cards have literally changed the way we go about our daily business.

Our conversations commonly allude to magnetism. We speak of someone's having a "magnetic personality." "Opposites attract" has become a tired cliché. We use them every day and talk about their properties, but have you ever wondered what makes a magnet a magnet?

If something attracts iron, it is a magnet. The ancients first noticed this property in naturally magnetic stones, composed of magnetite, a chemical compound of iron and oxygen. The word *magnet,* we're told, derives from the Greek word meaning "the stone of Magnesia," the ancient city where lodestone was first found.

Over time, other observations were made about these lodestones. At the end of the thirteenth century an Italian engineer, Peter Peregrinus, described their polarized nature in a letter to a friend. Sometimes two stones were drawn to each other, but when one was turned in the opposite direction, they pushed each other away. The lodestones also, noted Peregrinus, always faced in a north-south direction when floated in water.

MODERN MAGNETS

Although most of us think of magnets as being metallic, they can be made from other materials as well. Physicists tell us that what makes something magnetic has to do with unpaired spinning electrons. Some materials have an abundance of such electrons, and the atoms in these materials gather together in clusters called magnetic domains. Although each individual domain is a little magnet, the domains face in many different directions. When a strong magnetic field is applied to this unruly gang, they all align and spin in the same direction.

In modern times, we create magnets by applying a large, brief pulse of direct current to a coil of wire. This, in turn, produces a very strong magnetic field, which aligns the domains of a magnetizable substance placed in or near the coil. Once this happens, we have a magnet.

TEMPORARY VERSUS PERMANENT MAGNETS

Some combinations of metals (alloys) are easily magnetized but lose their magnetism when the magnetic field is removed. One such alloy of nickel and iron, Permalloy, is used as a temporary magnet in telephones and electric motors.

Other alloys retain their magnetic properties and make very good permanent magnets. Those most commonly used for making permanent healing magnets (biomagnets) are the ferrites—ceramic-like materials composed of iron oxides combined with nickel, cobalt, barium, or other metals. To make flexible biomagnets that easily wrap around a body part, manufacturers combine a ferrite mixture with plastic, rubber, or other pliable materials. An alloy of iron and boron combined with the rare-earth element neodymium makes the strongest permanent biomagnet, since this material is able to hold more magnetism.

MEASURING MAGNETIC FIELDS

Do you remember the grade school science experiment in which your teacher placed a piece of paper with iron filings over a horseshoe magnet? The filings accumulated mostly at the north and south poles of the horseshoe. These were the areas where there were more lines of magnetic flux.

Measuring the number of magnetic flux lines is the way scientists commonly assess the power of a biomagnet. The unit of measure used is called a gauss, named after German astronomer and mathematician Carl Friedrich Gauss. Another unit used to measure magnetic flux density is tesla, named after Nikola Tesla, who invented the alternating-current (AC) electrical system. (One tesla = 10,000 gauss.) Scientists use extremely sensitive instruments called gaussmeters or magnetometers to measure magnetic fields.

THE MAGNETIC EARTH

About four hundred years ago, an English scientist and physician to Queen Elizabeth I, William Gilbert, cut a piece of lodestone into the shape of a ball and put tiny pieces of iron all over it. He discovered that the iron lined up in the same way that compass needles did at various places on the earth. The earth, he concluded, was a magnetized ball.

Gilbert was indeed right. The center of the earth is a large, very strong magnet. By the time this magnetic field reaches the earth's surface, however, it becomes rather weak—only about .5 gauss. The earth's surface magnetism is strongest at two points—one near the geographic north pole and one near the geographic south pole. These two areas have the densest concentration of magnetic flux lines.

The spinning of hot molten iron at the earth's core produces its magnetic field. The earth also has an electric field caused by the action of high-energy ultraviolet light coming from the sun, which creates charged particles (ions) in the ionosphere. The earth's magnetic field is far from static. It fluctuates in response to changes in the ionic atmosphere, the most dramatic action being the magnetic storms caused by solar flares. The earth's magnetic field also changes as the moon revolves around it. And scientists have discovered that the earth's poles have actually reversed themselves many times, although it takes at least 10,000 years—and more typically 100,000 to 1 million years—for such shifts to occur.[1]

THE BODY MAGNETIC

About twenty-five years ago, Richard P. Blakemore, a graduate student at the University of Massachusetts, discovered that some bacteria contain one or more chains of magnetite particles—the original lodestone. In tracking their movements, he found that these minuscule mineral crystals acted as compass needles, guiding these simple creatures along geomagnetic field lines.

Since then, magnetite has also been found in a diverse range of more complex animals, including pigeons, salmon, honeybees, turtles, and dolphins. And in 1983, R. Robin Baker, a University of Manchester researcher, succeeded in locating magnetic deposits in the human brain, close to the pituitary and pineal glands.[2]

In one experiment, in which high school students were blindfolded and earmuffed, the ones who had a magnet in their headbands were unable to sense direction correctly, whereas those who had brass bars in their headbands maintained their sense of direction.[3] It now appears that sensing direction magnetically may be common to all living creatures—from the simplest to the most complex.

The pineal gland, located in the center of the brain, has been found to be affected by even very small magnetic fields. Melatonin, the hormone secreted by this sensitive gland, is involved not only in "fine-tuning" biological rhythms but in many other physiological functions as well. Scientists are now finding evidence that seasonal affective disorder (winter depression), which is associated with abnormal melatonin levels, may be the result not only of decreased light in the winter but also of changes in the earth's magnetic field.[4] The gland's sensitivity to these fields may explain the jump in psychiatric hospitalizations after magnetic storms that Dr. Robert O. Becker observed so many years ago.

Further evidence of the body's magnetic field has been provided by the results of an experiment performed by psychobiologist Dr. John Zimmerman, president of the Bio-Electro Magnetics Institute (BEMI). While a faculty member at the University of Colorado School of Medicine, Zimmerman measured the body's magnetism using an instrument capable of detecting magnetic fields a billion times weaker than the earth's. He was able to document a distinct magnetic field emanating from an individual engaged in laying-on-of-hands healing. The field was also measurable when the healer was not treating a patient, and it was distinctly different than when the healer was working.[5]

Just as the earth has both magnetic and electrical fields, so does the human body. The body's tissues contain charged particles (ions). Some common examples are positively charged sodium, calcium, and potassium ions and negatively charged chloride, which are found both within our cells and in the fluid that surrounds them. The constant motion of these charged particles, which underlies all of our physiological functions, creates both electrical and magnetic fields.

Magnetism and electricity are intimately related forces. Moving electric charges produce magnetic fields. And magnetic fields exert forces on moving electric charges. These basic principles were used in designing the magnetic resonance imaging (MRI) machine. The strong magnetic field applied to the body aligns all of its positively charged hydrogen atoms in the same direction. The subsequent application of radio waves and computer translation of the ions' movement allows the detailed imaging of body organs.

ELECTROMAGNETIC SMOG

So here we are: amazingly complex electromagnetic beings living on the earth and interacting with its dynamic fields. We have made things even more complicated by creating new technologies that emit additional fields. A hundred years ago, the only electromagnetic fields with which we interacted were the earth's field, visible light, and periodic lightning. Since then, we have filled our atmosphere with shortwaves, radio and television waves, microwaves, and more.

Our homes and offices are furnished with equipment and appliances that are electrically powered by alternating current, which continually changes direction. The electric field changes from plus to minus, and the magnetic field alternates between north and south. In the United States and most of the Northern Hemisphere, this field changes direction 120 times a second, completing 60 cycles per second. AC current in Europe and the former Soviet Union completes 50 cycles per second. Scientists characterize such current frequencies in terms of hertz, named after the German scientist Heinrich Hertz, who first studied this phenomenon (for example, a frequency of 60 cycles per second = 60 hertz).

The evidence is mounting that these 50- to 60-hertz electromagnetic fields adversely affect our biological systems. If you've found yourself feeling irritated or fatigued after working at a computer all day, you're not alone. The Swedes call this "electrical hypersensitivity" and have noted symptoms that, in addition to the aforementioned, include headaches, dizziness, nausea, and skin rashes.

The Swedes also examined the effects of 50-hertz electromagnetic fields on more than half a million people. The results, reported by researchers in 1995, showed a definite relationship between childhood leukemia and proximity to electrical power lines.[6] American researchers have found that 60-hertz fields interfere with the pineal gland and melatonin's ability to block the growth of breast cancer cells.[7] Such findings have led the Environmental Protection Agency (EPA) to investigate not only the polluted water table but also exposure to 60-hertz fields as causal factors in the extremely high incidence of breast cancer among New York women residing on Long Island.[8]

A number of researchers who presented studies in 1997 at the Second World Congress for Electricity and Magnetism in Biology and Medicine reported disrupting effects of 50- and 60-hertz fields not only on the pineal gland but also on the thymus and thyroid glands.[9] Our bodies' metabolism and immune response depend on the health of these very important endocrine glands. Their inefficient functioning can lead to a wide variety of maladies.

In recent years, we've also been seeing a growing number of reports about the biological effects of mobile phones, which operate in the radio-wave megahertz range. European studies have noted symptoms such as fatigue, headaches,[10] and increased resting blood pressure[11] associated with mobile phone use. In one German study, researchers reported that the operation of a mobile telephone caused an increase in certain brain waves.[12] Other German researchers have noted that electromagnetic fields produced by mobile phones suppressed REM sleep—that deep, restorative stage of sleep essential for memory and learning processes.[13] Some animal studies suggest that radio-frequency fields accelerate the development of certain types of cancers, and one Russian researcher recently concluded that "long-term exposure (over one year) combined with the organism-weakened immune system may produce a cumulative effect in the form of stress responses, various damages and, in some cases, even cancer."[14]

BEING OUT OF SYNC

Scientists who have looked at the earth's natural fields and human brain waves are providing us with some clues as to why our everyday electrical current is causing untoward physiological effects.

All magnetic fields involve the movement of charged particles. These fields can be produced from either direct current (DC) or alternating current. Zimmerman uses the image of a river flowing downhill to describe unidirectional direct current. A DC magnetic field is known as a static field because it stays steady and does not switch polarities back and forth. DC magnetic fields exist not only around DC power lines but also around lodestones (natural magnets) or around man-made magnets.

Alternating current, in contrast, switches back and forth between a plus and a minus electric field, producing a magnetic field that alternates between north and south. "Think of it like an ocean tide moving in and out," says Zimmerman. With the AC electricity we use in the United States, the electrons move in and out 120 times each second, completing 60 cycles (60 hertz).

It turns out that the earth has both DC and AC electromagnetic fields. A DC static field of about .5 gauss exists at the earth's surface. In the 1960s, the National Bureau of Standards detected AC electromagnetic fields superimposed on the DC static field. These Schumann waves (named after the physicist who first proposed their existence) have frequencies ranging from about 8 cycles per second (8 hertz) to 32 cycles per second (32 hertz), with the most predominant of these frequency peaks being the 8-hertz ones. The magnetic field of 8 hertz is in the nanotesla to picotesla range (a billionth or a trillionth tesla). If you're like me, that's really difficult to imagine, so I like to describe it as Zimmerman does—"way beyond very tiny."

Interestingly, when human brain-wave frequencies are measured by electroencephalograms (EEGs), they are found to range from .5 to 30 hertz. The 8-hertz Schumann frequency, in fact, is the very same frequency as the slower end of an alpha brain wave (8 to 12 hertz). Alpha brain waves are predominant when we close our eyes and are also common during meditation and other states of deep relaxation.

Alpha brain waves have been associated with good health. Researchers have documented that people who are meditators and regularly spend time in the alpha state are healthier than their nonmeditating peers.[15] Intriguing research conducted by Dr. Robert C. Beck found a brain-wave frequency of 7.8 to 8.0 hertz occurring in energy healers, regardless of their discipline or belief systems (Christian faith healers, Hawaiian kahunas,

Wicca practitioners, and so forth), when they entered an altered state of consciousness to do their work.[16]

Although being in sync with the earth's 8-hertz frequency appears to be conducive to good health, we are chronically exposed to frequencies that are nearly eight times as fast as the earth's most predominant frequency. The alternating magnetic field created by a 50- to 60-hertz current is about .03 gauss—much larger than the "way beyond very tiny" magnetic field of an 8-hertz frequency. Radio waves and microwaves, in the million- and billion-hertz range, are even further out of sync with the earth's natural AC fields.

The brain houses the pituitary and pineal glands. Because these neuroendocrine glands are involved in a myriad of regulatory activities that maintain a healthy balance in our bodies, we begin to get an inkling of why our man-made electromagnetic fields can impact our well-being in such a variety of ways.

Although chronic exposure to AC electromagnetic fields with frequencies higher than our bodies' brain waves can harm us, static magnetic fields, in which the field doesn't fluctuate (frequency = 0), are being found to be beneficial for healing and restoring balance. At this point in time, we do know a bit more than the ancients did when they discovered that static magnets were effective healing tools. We'll explore some of the current thinking about how they work in chapter 4.

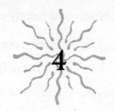

4

How Magnets Heal

Although we gain a bit more knowledge each year about how magnets work, we are still very much in a learning curve. Currently, many different theories have been proposed to explain the mechanisms underlying the healing results we see.

THE POLE STORY

Before we can explore the latest thinking on the issue, however, we need to get clear on the naming conventions used for healing magnets (biomagnets). Biomagnet scientists, practitioners, and manufacturers, it turns out, have a language all their own. And unless we understand their terminology, we'll feel as if we were wandering aimlessly in the Tower of Babel.

North and South

Let's start with how magnet poles are named traditionally and in the biomagnet world. In the traditional scientific-industrial-maritime world, the end of a magnet that points toward the geographic north pole of the earth is named the "north pole," and the end that points toward the geographic south pole is named the "south pole."

The biomagnetic way of naming poles is completely the opposite. In the biomagnetic convention, the north pole of a magnet is the end that is attracted toward the south geographical pole, where the south magnetic pole of the earth is also located. The south pole of the magnet is the end that is attracted toward the north geographical pole, where the earth's magnetic north pole is located. With biomagnets, we think about the north pole's being "south-seeking" and the south pole's being "north-seeking."

Negative and Positive

Another biomagnetic naming convention labels the north pole "negative" and the south pole "positive." This labeling is based on the fact that a biomagnetic north pole moves the needle of a magnetometer (a magnetic measuring device) toward the left, or negative, side of the scale, whereas a biomagnetic south pole moves the needle to the right, or positive, side of the scale. In the biomagnetic world, the terms *north* and *negative*, and *south* and *positive* are often used interchangeably in talking about the different healing effects of each pole.

Unipolar and Bipolar

The other two terms we need to be familiar with to understand the "hows" of magnet therapy are *unipolar* and *bipolar*. Unipolar refers to a healing magnet that is designed in such a way that only one pole of the magnet—either north *or* south (but not both)—faces the body, while the opposite pole faces away from the body. Most unipolar magnet therapy uses the north pole facing the body and the south pole facing away.

Bipolar refers to a healing magnet that is designed so that both poles—north *and* south—face the body. Both unipolar and bipolar magnets are commonly available in the marketplace, and beneficial results have been reported from using both types. As you will see, the "pole story" is very much connected to the "how magnets work" story.

HOW MAGNETS WORK

We know from research studies, clinical experience, and thousands of anecdotal reports that magnet therapy relieves pain, speeds healing, and appears to restore balance when our systems get out of whack. Nobody is really sure how this comes about, but let's look at some of the theories proposed by scientists and experienced magnet therapists.

To Relieve Pain

The experts offer a couple of different theories about how magnets might relieve pain.

ELECTRICAL POTENTIAL

Vincent Ardizonne, the designer of a checkerboard-pattern bipolar magnet, proposes that bipolar magnets alter the nerve cells (neurons) in such a way that sensation of pain is blocked.

Whether it's pain resulting from a chronic condition or an acute injury, the pain signal is transmitted from one neuron to another, first to the spinal cord and then to the brain. This transmission involves a change in the electrical potential of the nerve cells (the difference in the electrical charge between the inside and the outside of the cells).

According to Ardizonne, magnets induce a voltage in the neurons so that their normal resting electrical potential is maintained and the transmission of pain impulses is prevented. For a person to feel pain, the impulses must move to the brain, where the pain centers are located. If the impulses don't move, there will be no perception of pain.

ENDORPHINS

Another theory has to do with endorphins, the body's natural pain relievers. These small protein molecules have a structure that is very similar to morphine. The term *endorphins*, in fact, means endogenous (internally created) morphines. Like morphine, they attach to opiate receptors in the brain and other body cells, creating an analgesic effect.

Endorphin levels have been demonstrated to increase with vigorous exercise ("runner's high"), and they are related to moods. Positive thoughts and feelings increase their levels, whereas people who are unhappy have lower levels. It has also been documented that endorphins are released during needle acupuncture and that this is one of the mechanisms behind acupuncture's ability to relieve pain.[1]

Acupuncture analgesia can be quite dramatic. Many of us remember watching television footage in the early 1970s of fully conscious patients in China who underwent surgery painlessly—with only a few inserted acupuncture needles.

Now, we have evidence that magnets also increase endorphin levels in the body. Dr. Saul Liss, a biomedical engineer who, along with his brother, has invented a number of FDA-approved electromagnetic devices, presented very interesting findings at the 1999 meeting of the North American Academy of Magnetic Therapy. Liss reported that two hours after treatment with a static magnet on a particular acupuncture point, the endorphin level had increased 48 percent from its pretreatment level.[2]

Given that there are approximately two thousand acupuncture points on the body,[3] it seems likely that even when a biomagnet is not intentionally placed on an acupuncture point, there would be contact with one or more points and that the magnetic field would act to increase pain-relieving endorphins. As acupuncture has been found to stimulate the immune system as well as increase neurotransmitters and neurohormones, magnetic contact with these points may also enhance healing and contribute to the restoration of balance within the body.

To Speed Healing

It is believed that magnets accelerate the healing process primarily through increasing blood flow into the capillaries—the tiny permeable blood vessels that allow for the transfer of oxygen, water, and glucose from the blood into the cells. Increased blood flow in response to magnet therapy has been documented by European researchers[4] and by magnet therapists, such as neurologist Dr. Ron Lawrence, in unpublished studies.[5]

Physicists say this is a combined result of the Hall effect and Faraday's law. With bipolar magnets, the scientists explain, billions of charged particles within the blood vessels whiz back and forth, banging the left and then the right sides of the vessels in response to the alternating spatial pattern of north and south magnetic poles in a bipolar magnet. This results in heat and an increase in the diameter of the blood vessels (vasodilation), allowing more blood to move through the vessels. Others think that the increase in circulation has to do with the fact that the blood contains oxygen-binding hemoglobin and that the iron component of hemoglobin is responsive to the application of a magnetic field.

Regardless of why it happens, the increased blood flow brings more nutrients and oxygen to the injured area. At the same time, it accelerates the movement of specialized cells called phagocytes. Phagocytes are essential to the healing process, as they remove debris, repair tissue, and counteract the inflammatory chemicals that cause pain.

To Restore Balance

There are a variety of theories as to how magnetic fields might restore the body's natural state of balance. Let's take a look at a few of them.

BLOOD PH

The pH is a measure of the alkalinity or acidity of a solution, with a scale ranging from 0 to 14. The lower the number, the more acidic the solution, with 7.0 being neutral. The normal pH of the blood is slightly alkaline, at 7.4.

According to physician and longtime magnet therapist Dr. William Philpott, normal physiological processes and wellness are dependent on the maintenance of an alkaline pH. Stress and a meat-based diet are just two of the factors that can tip the body's acid-base balance. According to Philpott, "Allergies, intolerances, chemical hypersensitivities, insect stings and most toxins are acids or biologically acid evoking."[6] Fungi, bacteria, and parasites, notes Philpott, thrive in an acidic environment.

Philpott claims his clinical experience supports the research done by Dr. Albert Roy Davis and Walter C. Rawls that negative (north) pole magnetic energy promotes tissue alkalinity, whereas positive (south) pole magnetic energy promotes tissue acidity.[7] According to Philpott, the application of negative alkalinizing magnetic energy supports biological healing by oxygenating tissues, reducing inflammation and edema, relieving pain, fighting infection, and restoring normal cell metabolism.

CALCIUM

Psychologist and magnet therapy researcher Dr. Buryl Payne proposes that magnetic fields affect the migration of calcium ions. The calcium is moved to where it is needed—say, to speed the healing of a broken bone—and moved away from where it is damaging, such as arthritic joints and clogged blood vessels. A study recently conducted at Hunter College in New York confirmed that calcium plays a role in the response of cells to electromagnetic fields.[8]

ELECTRON TRANSFER

Dentist Dr. Dean R. Bonlie, founder of the Advanced Magnetic Research Institute (AMRI) in Calgary, Canada, and the inventor of the Magnetic Molecular Energizing (MME) device, proposes that our cells lose their normal charge from the stress of daily living, including exposure to 60-hertz electromagnetic fields. He proposes that they can be restored to a healthy state by exposure to a negative (north pole) magnetic field. Bonlie holds that negative magnetic fields increase the speed at which electrons move, resulting in enhanced electron transfer. These accelerated electrons, according to Bonlie, enhance chemical reactions in the body, leading to improvement in all functions.

Bonlie cites scientific evidence of the measurement of the earth's magnetic field that shows that its strength has decreased tenfold over the last four thousand years.[9] He also supports Dr. Kyoichi Nakagawa's magnetic deficiency syndrome theory.

Director of the Isuzu Hospital in Tokyo, Nakagawa has spent more than twenty years researching the effects of magnetism on humans. He notes that metal buildings and vehicles absorb the earth's magnetic energy and concludes that spending our days in steel-supported buildings and metal vehicles limits our exposure to the earth's natural magnetic field.

Our modern style of living, according to Nakagawa, can lead to magnetic deficiency syndrome, characterized by such symptoms as chronic fatigue, insomnia, headaches, dizziness, and a whole host of aches and pains. The way to reverse or prevent the syndrome is to ensure that the body has adequate direct-current magnetism.[10] This can be achieved through restoring the field with magnetic devices—mattresses, pads, jewelry, and so forth.

ENZYMES

Enzymes are proteins that act as catalysts to speed up chemical reactions in the body. Every cell in the body produces enzymes, which have very specialized functions. Pancreas cells, for example, produce lipase, protease, and amylase, which are needed for the efficient digestion of different types of food. The liver produces many enzymes, which perform different jobs. Some break down fats, while others are involved in the detoxification process. Every function in the body is dependent on enzyme activity.

We know that enzymes are influenced by many factors, and psychobiologist Dr. John Zimmerman proposes that magnets may beneficially affect enzyme activity. His view is supported by numerous studies, including the work of biochemist Dr. Justa Smith. Smith confirmed earlier findings that magnetic fields accelerated the reaction rate of various enzymes. She then went on to prove that the magnetic energy emitted from the hands of energy healers could also impact the reaction rates of enzymes.[11] According to an unpublished report from the Department of Biology of Guangdong College of Education in China, even magnetized water can quicken enzyme reaction rates.[12]

SEROTONIN

Serotonin is a neurotransmitter. It biochemically transmits a signal from one nerve cell (neuron) to another across the space between neurons, called a synapse. Most serotonin is in the neurons, but it is also found in other body tissues. Serotonin influences many parts of the brain and many physiological functions, including behavior, mood, pain, movement, cardiovascular function, endocrine secretion, appetite, and sexuality. Low levels have been associated with mood disorders, depression, insomnia, anxiety, bulimia, anorexia, migraine headaches, and decreased pain tolerance.

In the same presentation in which he reported an increase in endorphins after treatment with magnet therapy, Liss also reported that there was a significant increase in serotonin in the people he studied. He postulates that blood flowing in a magnetic field can generate a current in nerves and that this current adds to the current already in the nerve. This increase in energy would result in the body's production of more serotonin and other needed biochemicals. He supports his theory with the facts that electromagnetic therapy with his devices has had positive effects on all of the aforementioned conditions and that he has measured increased serotonin levels after treatment. He feels that magnetic energy "facilitates the body to help itself."[13]

WATER

The bodies of all living organisms are composed mostly of water. Overall, the human body is about 70 percent water, and some structures, like the brain, contain 80 percent water. Some scientists think that the overall balancing effects of magnets are related to the changes in the structure of water within the body.

The exact mechanism by which this happens is not yet clear. However, we do know that when a magnetic field is applied to water, molecular water clusters separate. This changes the surface tension of the water, allowing it to be more easily absorbed.

Experiments conducted on plants provide some evidence that magnetized water does have an effect. As noted in chapter 2, researchers have shown that seedlings watered with magnet-treated water had a 68 percent germination rate compared to the 8 percent germination rate of tap-watered seedlings.[14] Results of a pilot study conducted recently at the Vegetable Improvement Center of Texas A&M University revealed that squash plants grown with magnetically treated spring water were heavier and produced heavier vegetables than those grown with untreated spring water.[15]

In humans, magnetized water has been shown to increase enzyme reaction time[16] and to be effective in treating intestinal parasitic disease in children.[17]

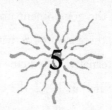

5

Looking at the Evidence

THE NEW MEDICINE

Everyone would agree that we are in the midst of a medical revolution in America. More than 40 percent of us, according to a recent nationwide study by Harvard researchers, are using alternative therapies not currently incorporated into mainstream medicine.[1] And physicians, once considered the ultimate source of medical information, now often find their patients more knowledgeable about natural, nontoxic remedies than they are.

Because most of our physicians don't know much about alternative and complementary therapies, we've been educating ourselves. With easy access through the Internet, we can read the same medical journals they do. The problem is that very little alternative medicine research finds its way into peer-reviewed journals archived in the National Library of Medicine database.

Wait, you say. Isn't the government now funding alternative medicine research? Yes, there is some activity. Originally founded as the Office for Alternative Medicine within the National Institutes of Health (NIH) in 1992, the office has recently been elevated in status to the National Center for Complementary and Alternative Medicine (NCCAM), and research funding has been increasing year after year. From the $5 million allocation in 1992, the budget had grown to $50 million by fiscal year 1998. Although this is a tenfold increase, it is still only 1.5 percent of the total funds set aside for NIH research.

Medical research in this country is driven by pharmaceutical and high-tech interests. As consumers continue to push for natural healing approaches, I am hopeful that research into alternative and complementary therapies will increase. However, given the entrenchment of the powers that be and the financial stakes involved, this increase is likely to be inch by inch rather than mile by mile.

In the meantime, I believe we need to look at other sources of evidence as the Europeans do. In Germany, for example, the government established Commission E in 1978 to regulate botanical (herbal) remedies. The government agency's evaluation process doesn't limit itself to evidence from well-designed human studies. It also considers traditional usage experience when deciding whether or not to approve a submitted remedy for over-the-counter sale.

MAGNET THERAPY EVIDENCE

If we only look at peer-reviewed journal articles, we will be missing a lot of valuable information. This is particularly the case with magnet therapy. Magnet therapy is an accepted healing modality in many European and Asian countries, where pharmaceuticals play a far less prominent role than they do in the United States. Much of the research from these countries isn't translated into English, but when we can gain access to it, it is definitely worth examining. For example, family practice physician Dr. William Pawluk and Dr. Jiri Jerabek, former director of the National Institute of Public Health in the Czech Republic, recently compiled an English translation of 343 studies conducted on magnet therapy during the last thirty years in Eastern Europe.

Some magnet manufacturers fund their own research. These investigations can be well-designed studies carried out in respected clinical settings. Again, this information, available from manufacturers, isn't published in established journals. However, it, too, I feel, is worthy of review. The results, of course, may be biased because of the vested interest of the manufacturer—but probably no more or no less than the drug research in this country, which is primarily funded by pharmaceutical companies.

Observations of magnet therapy practitioners are yet another valuable source of information, as are the experiences of people like you and me, who have reached for magnets to treat ailments and have found them helpful. Alth observations are not as scientifically valid as systematic evaluations, repeated reports build a body of valuable, real-life information that shouldn't be dismissed. Most people don't realize that only 10 to 20 percent of mainstream treatments used in this country have undergone rigorous clinical trials.[2]

In examining the evidence compiled in this chapter, I invite you to be as open-minded as Paracelsus, who searched for the truth from many sources: learned physicians, experts, wise women, alchemists, nobles, clergy, lay healers—and the common folk.

RESEARCH DESIGN

Since researchers have a language all their own, let me clarify a few terms before we go further. *Placebo-controlled* refers to a study in which one group of patients (the treatment group) is given a "real" treatment while another group (the control group) is given a "fake" or "sham" treatment. This type of study design attempts to eliminate the concern that changes in patients' conditions are due solely to any intervention—the "placebo effect." In most placebo-controlled studies, patients are randomly assigned to either a treatment group or a control group.

The term *double-blind* refers to a study in which neither the patients nor the researchers know whether the treatment is real or sham. This type of study design attempts to control for bias that may occur when this information is known.

A *crossover* study design is one in which both the treatment group and the control group switch roles, so that each patient in the study participates in a treatment group and a control group.

To achieve the highest degree of scientific objectivity, researchers often incorporate more than one element into their study designs.

MAGNET THERAPY STUDIES

Wherever I could find evidence regarding static magnets, I present those findings. However, since there is currently only a very small body of static magnet research and most of the published research regarding magnet therapy is about pulsed (on-and-off) electromagnetic fields (PEMFs) or other alternating-current (AC) therapy, I include some of these latter studies as well. In some areas with extensive electromagnetic literature, I present only a sampling of representative studies due to space limitations.

Although extrapolation from PEMF and other AC studies provides implications for static bipolar magnet therapy, it's not quite an exact fit. As you may recall from chapter 3, with AC current, the electrical field switches back and forth from positive to negative. As the electrical field varies, the magnetic field associated with the current fluctuates between north and south polarity. With bipolar static magnets, both north and south polarities are applied to the body at the same time, and there is no time interruption in the application of the field as there is with pulsed therapy.

Experts such as Pawluk, psychobiologist Dr. John Zimmerman, and biomedical engineer Dr. Saul Liss have noted that both AC electromagnetic treatments and stationary magnets have beneficial effects but that the healing is quicker with AC treatments. For example, Liss found that both static magnetic fields and AC electromagnetic fields produced similar increases in endorphins, neurotransmitters, and certain hormones. Whereas it took two hours to produce these results with a static magnet, it took only twenty minutes with an electromagnetic device.[3]

When I reviewed the electromagnetic studies, I found that there was a wide variation in the strength of the magnetic field, the frequency of the AC current, the interval between pulses, and the length and frequency of treatments used. The answers as to what are the very best treatment protocols for various conditions have not yet emerged. Similar questions also have not yet been answered for stationary magnets. Although we're not concerned with current frequencies with static magnets, some of the hottest issues are whether bipolar or unipolar magnets are more effective or whether certain conditions would respond more favorably to one type of magnet or the other.

CONDITIONS FOR WHICH
MAGNET THERAPY HAS BEEN FOUND HELPFUL

Even though there are still unanswered questions, the exciting news is that many people with a wide range of ailments are benefiting from magnet therapy. Let's now take a look at some of the conditions for which it has been found helpful.

Back, Neck, and Shoulder Pain

In a Japanese study, 121 patients with severe chronic shoulder pain were treated with static magnets at the Hospital of Kinki University and the Hospital of Tokyo Medical College. Of those treated with higher-strength magnets, 82 percent reported a significant improvement in pain, whereas 37 percent of those treated with a lower-strength magnet showed improvement within four days.[4] Dr. Kyoichi Nakagawa (developer of the magnetic field deficiency syndrome theory), who has treated more than 11,000 patients with static magnets, has reported a 90 percent success rate in patients whose primary complaints were neck, shoulder, and back pain.[5]

A double-blind, placebo-controlled study of one hundred patients conducted in the Orthopedic Department of the Klinic Bavaria found static magnets effective in relieving lower back, neck, and shoulder pain. Of those treated with magnet therapy for fourteen days, 70 percent experienced a reduction in pain. In contrast, 26 percent of the group receiving sham treatment reported a decrease in pain symptoms.[6]

Here in the United States, Zimmerman and Dr. Edward Collacott, division chief of the Physical Medicine Department at the Veterans Administration Medical Center in Prescott,

Arizona, are conducting a double-blind, placebo-controlled, crossover study on the effect of static magnets on lower-back pain. This is the first placebo-controlled study to compare the effectiveness of both unipolar and bipolar magnets in relieving back pain.[7]

There is also evidence on the electromagnetic front. Irish researchers who conducted a double-blind, placebo-controlled study of patients with persistent neck pain found that pulsed electromagnetic therapy significantly decreased pain and improved range of movement.[8]

Compelling new electromagnetic evidence comes from American researchers. University of Texas Southwestern Medical Center scientists have recently published the results of their three-year investigation of percutaneous electrical nerve stimulation (PENS) for relief of acute low-back pain in the *Journal of the American Medical Association*. The device used is similar to the one used for transcutaneous electrical nerve stimulation (TENS), which has long been a proven pain relief modality. Rather than using electrode pads like TENS, PENS uses acupuncture-like needles, which allow results to be achieved with a lower, more comfortable electric current. After three to four PENS treatments, patients noted significant improvement in pain, activity, sleep, and the need for pain medication. The researchers are currently investigating the use of PENS for the treatment of neck pain, headaches, and diabetic neuropathy.[9]

Bone Fractures

In this country, several electromagnetic devices have been approved by the Food and Drug Administration (FDA) for treating bone fractures. Their beneficial effects—including the healing of long-standing, recalcitrant (nonunion) fractures—have been increasingly documented in medical journals since 1973.[10]

Both electromagnetic and static magnetic fields were shown to accelerate the healing of fractures in a number of animal studies conducted in Eastern Europe.[11] Favorable results were also seen in Eastern European human studies. In one study of fifty patients with wrist (Colles) fractures, researchers treated twenty-eight of those individuals electromagnetically, whereas twenty-two patients received sham treatments. After seven weeks, the fracture lines were not seen in those who had received magnet therapy, whereas the lines were still visible in all those in the control group.[12] In another Eastern European study, in which both electromagnetic and static fields were used, all treated patients experienced an analgesic effect and edema (swelling) reduction; however, the best results for forearm and hip fractures were obtained with static magnets.[13]

Carpal Tunnel Syndrome

An interim clinical report presented at the 1997 Second World Congress for Electricity and Magnetism in Biology and Medicine described a placebo-controlled, double-blind study in which static magnets were taped over the carpal tunnel of wrists of turkey plant workers. The researchers concluded that the device was side effect—free and effective in alleviating carpal tunnel pain.[14]

Jerabek and Pawluk included in their book a summary of an Eastern European study in which the use of static magnets was compared to the use of hydrocortisone cream in patients with carpal tunnel syndrome. Of the 119 patients who were treated with static magnets, a good or an excellent effect was reported for 55 percent who received twenty treatments, each lasting twenty minutes. The researchers concluded that the improvement in median nerve conductivity (the condition involves pressure on the nerve, which slows conductivity) in the magnet-treated patients was comparable to those treated with hydrocortisone cream.[15]

Very favorable results for carpal tunnel syndrome have been reported by the president of the North American Academy of Magnetic Therapy, neurologist Dr. Ron Lawrence. Lawrence measured the nerve transmission times in twenty-two patients who had mild or moderate carpal tunnel syndrome. He then had his patients wear magnets on their wrists for six to twelve weeks. When he measured nerve transmission times, he found them improved in 91 percent of his patients.[16]

Dental Problems

A recent American double-blind crossover study of twenty-nine patients, conducted by researchers at the College of Dental

Medicine, Medical University of South Carolina, Charleston, evaluated the effects of a magnetized water irrigator on plaque, calculus (tartar), and gum health. Irrigation with magnetized water resulted in 64 percent less calculus than nonmagnetized irrigation. However, the reduction in plaque, the precursor of tartar, was minimal. The researchers concluded, "The magnetized water oral irrigator could be a useful adjunct in the prevention of calculus accumulation in periodontal patients."[17]

One Eastern European researcher reported beneficial results of applying static magnets either on the face surface or within the mouth of patients with gingivitis (gum inflammation) or periodontal (tooth supporting structures) disease. After seven days of treatment, edema and newly developed vessels were reduced, and there were signs of collagen production—an indication of connective tissue growth. After fourteen to fifteen days, an anti-inflammatory effect was noted, with a reduction in the number of pathogenic microorganisms in the mouth.[18]

Another study of periodontal disease patients, conducted by Eastern European researchers, found that that those patients who had magnets attached to the skin over the area where their gums were inflamed experienced less pain, and quicker and less troublesome recovery after oral surgery, than did those who were given sham magnets.[19]

Both static magnet and electromagnetic treatment have been found helpful in the treatment of periodontal disease. In comparing the two modalities, an Eastern European researcher noted that both static magnet– and electromagnetic-treated patients showed reductions in inflammation after treatment. The anti-inflammatory effect, however, was more pronounced in those patients treated electromagnetically, and unlike the static magnet group, there were some beneficial effects as well on hardening of tissue and other disease symptoms.[20]

An American researcher has investigated the ability of electromagnetic therapy to accelerate healing after oral surgery. In addition to conventional therapy, a group of patients received pulsed electromagnetic therapy three to five days prior to oral surgery and after surgery until they were released from the hospital. The control group, in contrast, received only conventional treatment. Patients treated with both therapies healed significantly faster than those who received only conventional treatment.[21]

Depression

In recent years, research has been emerging regarding the use of magnet therapy for alleviating depression. The technique, called transcranial magnetic stimulation (TMS), involves placing an electromagnetic copper coil on the cerebral cortex area of the scalp. A high-intensity current is rapidly turned on and off (pulsed), creating a strong magnetic field of 20,000 gauss—the same strength used in magnetic resonance imaging (MRI).

Researchers use repeated rhythmic stimulation, known as repetitive TMS (rTMS), with varied frequencies, with the pulse lasting usually for 100 to 200 microseconds.

In a study published in *Lancet* in 1996, Spanish researchers performed a placebo-controlled, multiple crossover study on seventeen patients with medication-resistant depression. Of the seventeen patients treated, eleven showed significant improvement after five days of daily rTMS sessions.[22]

Austrian researchers reported the results, in 1996, of a controlled study of TMS as an add-on therapy to standard antidepressive medications. The twelve patients enrolled in the study who received TMS in addition to medications had a greater remission of depressive symptoms than did the twelve enrolled patients who received only medications.[23]

A 1997 American study, conducted by researchers in the Department of Psychiatry at Emory University School of Medicine, treated fifty patients with rTMS for nonresponsive depression. Twenty-one of the fifty (42 percent) responded favorably to the therapy.[24]

In a 1997 placebo-controlled crossover trial, conducted by Dr. Mark S. George and colleagues at Medical University of South Carolina, depression was relieved in twelve patients when they received two weeks of rTMS treatment. In contrast, when the same patients underwent sham treatment for two weeks, their depression worsened.[25]

The mechanism for the beneficial effect of TMS on depression, according to scientists, is the depolarization of brain neurons. Although rTMS appears to be a potentially effective treatment for serious depression and a possible replacement for the more invasive and disruptive electroconvulsive therapy (ECT), the major safety concern is that the therapy has been known to induce seizures at fast frequencies. No seizures, however, have occurred when rTMS is delivered at a slow frequency of 1 hertz or less.[26] Two recent Israeli studies[27] and an American one[28] have verified the effectiveness of rTMS at slow frequencies.

Unfortunately, little information is available regarding using static magnets for treating depression. Dr. William Philpott, who has been involved with magnet therapy for a couple of decades, notes that "it appears from clinical observation that bitemporal placement [of negative pole magnets] usually is most appropriate for emotional and mental illnesses." He also states, "Depression, anxiety and panic are all likely to be helped by raising melatonin by sleeping with negative magnetic energy at the top of the head." "The crown of the head should rest 2 to 3 inches from the magnets," advises Philpott.[29]

Epilepsy

There are a few peer-reviewed studies about the effect of electromagnetic therapy on epilepsy. A German study recently published in *Lancet* describes a reduction in seizures in eight of nine patients treated with low-frequency rTMS therapy—the same type of treatment found beneficial for patients with severe recalcitrant depression.[30]

In a 1991 report of three patients with partial seizures, the authors indicated that the application of a low-intensity magnetic field resulted in a decrease in seizure frequency.[31] A 1992 case report, in which low-frequency electromagnetic therapy was also used, described decreased seizure frequency and a lessening of behavioral disturbances in a severe epileptic.[32]

Currently, a study using the same low-frequency (picotesla), low-level magnetic fields used by other researchers for successfully treating epilepsy is under way at the University of Oklahoma Health Sciences Center under the direction of Dr. Kalarickel Oommen. Preliminary observational reports are positive, indicating that seizure activity decreases in response to treatment.[33]

A couple of animal studies also provide supportive evidence. In one study, epilepsy was experimentally induced in rats. When modulated electromagnetic fields were administered, the seizures were suppressed.[34] In a recent study of mice, in which the rodents were pretreated with a static magnet, experimentally induced seizures were prevented.[35]

Based on clinical observations, some magnet therapists urge caution regarding self-treatment of epilepsy. Philpott, who outlines treatment for a wide range of conditions in his book

Biomagnetic Handbook, advises that treatment should only be carried out under close medical supervision.[36]

Dr. Ellen Kamhi (Ph.D., R.N.) is a multifaceted health practitioner who has been involved with electromagnetic healing for more than twenty years. Currently practicing at the Corsello Center for Integrative Medicine in Huntington, New York, Kamhi has seen the exacerbation of epileptic seizures in individuals who sleep on magnetic mattress pads. She cautions against the use of such mattresses by people with epilepsy.[37]

Fatigue

Other than the research on fibromyalgia (discussed later in the chapter), the only evidence we currently have about the ability of magnet therapy to relieve fatigue is anecdotal.

As I was researching this book, time and again I came across everyday people who told me that the static magnet products they were using—mattresses, pads, necklaces, insoles, and so on—were relieving fatigue.

A couple who do regular trade shows and have been wearing magnetic insoles during the shows told me that they noticed that their feet were less tired and that they were generally less depleted at the end of a demanding twelve-hour day. Others told me that they were able to exercise longer when they wore the insoles. A woman who had been sleeping on a magnetic mattress for a few weeks reported that she was sleeping less, dreaming more, and feeling more energetic upon awakening. A number of athletes who have been using magnets or drinking magnetized sports drinks claim increased endurance and improved performance. Hopefully, more research will be forthcoming in this area.

Female Problems

A number of studies support the use of magnet therapy for female problems, including painful menstruation (dysmenorrhea), endometriosis, chronic pelvic inflammatory disease (PID), and stress urinary incontinence.

In a placebo control-group study of twenty-three student nurses at South Korean University, researchers applied static magnets or sham magnets to young women suffering with menstrual pain. When pain assessments were made three hours after application of the magnets and three hours after removal of the magnets, the magnet-treated group reported significantly less pain than the sham-treated group.[38]

Eastern European researchers also report successful dysmenorrhea results from the application of static magnets. In this study, the magnets were applied to the pelvic area for three months during the second half of the menstrual cycle. Pain relief was achieved in 92.3 percent of those treated.[39] Kamhi has seen pain routinely relieved in her patients who apply static magnets to the pelvic area during their periods.[40]

Endometriosis, a condition in which the uterine lining (endometrium) overgrows, can cause heavy menstrual bleeding and severe back and abdominal pain. Eastern European researchers, in a number of studies, have found that the application of static magnets produced analgesia and also improved immune response in women suffering from endometriosis.[41] Researchers have also found magnetic-infrared-laser therapy combined with standard drug therapy to be effective in treating the condition.[42]

Italian researchers recently reported positive results from electromagnetic therapy for women suffering with pelvic pain for six months or longer. In this study, sixty-four women who had not responded to standard therapies were given electromagnetic treatment for two hours each day for twenty to forty days. When measures of pain reduction were taken three months after completion of the therapy, researchers found that the chronic pelvic pain had completely subsided in 61 percent. An additional 23 percent experienced complete relief from their pain during the treatment period; however, they had mild pelvic tension at three months posttreatment.[43]

Favorable results were also reported by Eastern European researchers in the treatment of chronic pelvic inflammatory disease (PID) with pulsed electromagnetic therapy. In 188 treated women, general improvement in both spontaneous and palpation (upon touching) pain was almost immediately noted. After the fourth to fifth exposure, 76 percent of the women experienced no palpation pain.[44]

Eastern European researchers have also investigated the use of magnet therapy for a number of other conditions, including reproduction function disturbances, gynecological inflammation, mammary fissures, and bartholin gland inflammation. One of the more intriguing findings was the alleviation of fallopian tube blockage in 98 of 115 women in response to electromagnetic therapy. With their tubes opened, 40 of the 98 successfully conceived.[45]

American researchers from Emory University School of Medicine recently reported success with the use of electromagnetic therapy for a common female problem—urinary stress incontinence. In this study, eighty-three women received stimulation to their pelvic floor muscles by sitting, fully clothed, on an electromagnetic seat. The study period lasted six weeks, during which the participants received twenty-minute sessions twice each week. A three-month follow-up found that 34 percent stayed continent and 32 percent used no more than one incontinence pad per day. Overall, daily pad usage dropped from 2.5 to 1.3, and the average number of leak episodes decreased from 3.3 to 1.7.[46]

Fibromyalgia

Fibromyalgia is a type of arthritis that currently afflicts 3.7 million Americans—mostly women. Its most common symptoms are chronic muscle pain in specific locales (tender points), fatigue, and insomnia. Manufacturers of magnetic mattresses claim that their products are helpful in alleviating the pain and fatigue associated with the condition, and many consumers have reported positive results.

Dr. Agatha Colbert reported the favorable results of a fibromyalgia–magnetic mattress study at the 1998 North American Magnetic Association meeting. In this double-blind, placebo-controlled study, conducted at Tufts Medical School, thirty fibromyalgia patients were given either magnetic or sham mattresses on which to sleep. Study subjects were not allowed any new treatments, such as medication, during the course of the study. Those in the magnetic group reported reduction in pain symptoms and improved sleep patterns, as well as a change in functional ability.[47]

Another controlled study has recently been completed at the University of Virginia's Center for the Study of Complementary and Alternative Therapies under the direction of Dr. Ann Gill Taylor (R.N., Ed.D., F.A.A.N.). Funded by NIH's National Center for Alternative and Complementary Medicine, the study of 116 patients explored the effect of a magnetic mattress as an adjunctive therapy for fibromyalgia.

Patients enrolled in the study continued with their medication regime and, in addition, were given a north unipolar mattress, a bipolar mattress, or a sham mattress to use for six months. Before-and-after measures looked at self-reports of sensory pain (how much it hurts) and affective pain (how bothersome it is). Changes in tender points and ability to function were also assessed.[48] As of this writing, a paper reporting the results of the study has been submitted for journal publication. Hopefully, it will provide useful information about the treatment of fibromyalgia and also shed some light on the unipolar versus bipolar effectiveness question.

Some clinical practitioners, like Kahmi, have found that people with fibromyalgia who sleep on magnetic mattresses experience relief from pain and fatigue for about two or three months but that the benefits fall off over time. Experts suspect that this type of response may be the result of the body's becoming used to the magnetic field and adapting to it (habituation). Kahmi recommends intermittent usage to prevent habituation.[49]

Foot Pain

A couple of recent American studies provide evidence that static magnets can be helpful in relieving certain types of foot pain. Intrigued by patients' telling him that magnets worked, neurologist Dr. Michael Weintraub decided to conduct a magnet therapy study on patients with peripheral neuropathy (nerve disease) of the feet—a condition that is generally unresponsive to conventional therapies.

Eight of the fourteen patients enrolled in the study had neuropathy caused by diabetes, whereas the other six had nondiabetic neuropathies. After four months of wearing 475-gauss magnetic insoles twenty-four hours a day, 75 percent of the diabetic patients reported a decrease in pain. In the nondiabetic group, 50 percent reported decreased pain.[50]

Weintraub followed up this study with a placebo-crossover one at New York Medical College in Briarcliff Manor. The patient population of twenty-four participants was randomly assigned to wear either magnetic (475-gauss) or sham insoles, and then the insoles were switched. Of the nineteen patients who completed the four-month study, ten had diabetic peripheral neuropathy, and nine had other painful neuropathies. In the diabetic group, 90 percent experienced reduced pain, whereas 33 percent of the nondiabetics reported relief of pain. Weintraub suspects that the variable response is related to a number of factors, including differences in nerve growth, damage, and metabolism between the two groups.[51]

Since pain returned when patients stopped using the insoles, Weintraub has concluded the treatment was "palliative but not curative." He is planning other studies on combining drug therapy with magnets for patients with peripheral neuropathy, foot tingling, and carpal tunnel syndrome.

Unpublished research conducted by podiatrist Dr. Larry Seaman at Barry University School of Podiatric Medicine in Miami, Florida, provides evidence for the beneficial use of static magnets for the treatment of heel spurs and other heel pain. In this double-blind, placebo-controlled study, twenty patients were provided with either magnetized or sham insoles. At the end of two weeks, 57.2 percent of those who had the magnetized insoles reported a subjective relief of pain, whereas 16.6 percent in the placebo group reported such relief. Improved walking was reported by 77.1 percent in the magnetized-sole group and by 16.6 percent of the placebo group.[52]

Headaches

A number of researchers have reported beneficial effects of pulsed electromagnetic therapy on headaches. Dr. Richard A. Sherman and his colleagues at the Madigan Army Medical Center in Tacoma, Washington, recently undertook two studies. In an open study, eleven patients with chronic migraine headaches were exposed to pulsing electromagnetic fields for one hour a day, five days per week. After two weeks, the number of weekly headaches decreased from 4.03 pretreatment to .43. A follow-up evaluation, an average of 8.1 months after treatment, revealed that the frequency of headaches had dropped even lower—to .14 per week.

The other study, conducted by these same researchers, was a double-blind one, in which nine patients were randomly assigned to either pulsed treatment or sham treatment for two weeks. The groups were then switched (crossovered). The frequency of headaches decreased on average from 3.32 to .58 per week in the study group.[53]

Dr. Reuven Sandyk, who has done a lot of work with picotesla (beyond very tiny) electromagnetic fields and the brain in treating a variety of neurological conditions, including Parkinson's disease and multiple sclerosis, has documented a successful treatment of a patient with acute migraine headaches by the application of picotesla electromagnetic fields.[54]

A paper presented at the 1987 Hungarian Symposium on Magnetotherapy documented that 88 percent of patients suffering from tension headaches had pain relief in response to treatment with electromagnetic fields. Patients with other types of headaches also responded favorably to the treatment—cervical migraines (68 percent) and migraines and psychogenic headaches (60 percent).[55]

In a paper presented at the same meeting, describing a double-blind, placebo-controlled study of the effects of pulsed electromagnetic fields on migraine headache patients, researchers noted that 66 percent of the treated patients obtained relief, in comparison to improvement in 23 percent of the placebo group.[56] Yet another presentation at the same meeting documented the success of pulsed electromagnetic therapy as a preventive treatment for patients with migraine and cervical headaches.[57]

Jerabek and Pawluk made note of two Eastern European studies using pulsed electromagnetic therapy to treat migraines. In one study, 60 percent of those treated showed a decrease in both intensity and frequency of headaches, whereas in the other study, 75 percent showed improvement.[58]

In a paper presented at a 1997 Russian symposium, researchers reported their successful treatment of 107 headache patients by exposing particular acupuncture points to an electromagnetic field from one of two devices. After three to five exposures, all patients experienced pain relief. A year later, 48 percent remained headache-free, and another 41 percent had a significant decrease in headaches.[59]

Evidence regarding headache treatment with static magnets is based on anecdotal reports and clinical observations. Kahmi, for example, has found static magnets to be effective in relieving headaches when they are applied to the area of the pain.[60] Philpott recommends placing a north-sided magnet directly over the painful area. If that doesn't relieve the pain, he suggests placing the magnet on the opposite side of the head. The third option he suggests is applying one magnet to each temple.[61]

High Blood Pressure

Static magnet therapy has been found to be helpful in bringing down elevated blood pressure (hypertension). Jerabek and Pawluk made note of two Eastern European studies in which hypertensive patients demonstrated decreased blood pressure after treatment with static magnets.[62]

In another Eastern European study, patients with moderate hypertension who had static magnets applied to their inner forearms for ten sessions of thirty to forty-five minutes' duration found relief from hypertensive symptoms such as dizziness, headache, and heart pain.[63]

Chinese-trained physician Dr. Xiu Ling Ma, currently a professor at Emperor's College of Traditional Oriental Medicine in Santa Monica, California, notes that static magnets are used in China to lower blood pressure in hypertensive patients and in the treatment of coronary artery disease. Research studies that support such treatments have been published in China.[64]

In this country, long-term magnet therapy practitioner Tom Nellessen reports the successful opening of blocked blood vessels as a result of wearing magnets. Some individuals who had been scheduled for coronary artery bypass surgery no longer required the operation, notes Nellessen. He attributes his own good heart health (despite a high-fat diet) to magnet therapy.[65]

Both static and electromagnetic fields have been demonstrated to be helpful in treating patients with moderate hypertension. Results of one Eastern European study, which used both static and electromagnetic fields to treat patients with moderate hypertension, indicated positive results from both types of treatment. In those who received treatment with static magnets, 68 percent improved, whereas in the group treated with electromagnetic therapy, 78 percent experienced beneficial results.[66]

Electromagnetic therapy, in a number of studies, has been found useful for treating not only hypertension but also other circulatory conditions, including ischemic heart disease and venous insufficiency. Intriguing preliminary data have recently been released about the ability of electromagnetic energy to regulate heart rates in dogs. Using the Jacobson Resonator, a device that emits low-level (picotesla) electromagnetic fields, University of Oklahoma Health Sciences Center scientists reported that they were able to cause either a slowing or a quickening of heart rate. Researchers Dr. Benjamin Scheriag and Dr. William Yamanashi are optimistic that these findings and their continuing research will lead to a new, noninvasive means for controlling heart rate and cardiovascular function in humans.[67]

Insomnia

Researchers have found electromagnetic low-energy emission therapy (LEET) to be effective in relieving chronic insomnia.[68] Colbert's report of the Tuft's University study of fibromyalgia patients (discussed in an earlier subsection) noted that the sleep patterns of those given magnetic mattresses improved. There are also many anecdotal reports claiming that sleeping on magnetic mattresses both improves the quality of sleep and decreases the amount of sleep needed.

Ma reports that magnet therapy is used in China for treating insomnia, restlessness, and irritability and that research has been published in China regarding such usage. From the Chinese medicine viewpoint, magnet therapy works in these conditions to calm the *shen*—the spiritual-emotional nature.[69]

Multiple Sclerosis

Multiple sclerosis is a degenerative condition of the central nervous system that can lead to severe debilitation. Mainstream medicine, as of yet, has not found a cure, but magnet therapy researchers are reporting results that offer promise for the many who suffer with this disease.

Most of the research in this country on using AC electromagnetic fields to treat multiple sclerosis has been undertaken by Dr. Reuven Sandyk. Sandyk's published reports are case studies describing the beneficial effects of very tiny, picotesla magnetic fields on various multiple sclerosis symptoms. Symptoms that have favorably responded in Sandyk's patients include fatigue, insomnia, vision, bowel and bladder function, movement, speech problems, mood, and cognitive function.[70]

Double-blind, placebo-controlled studies presented by researchers at the 1987 Hungarian Symposium on Magnetotherapy[71] and at the 1996 meeting of the European Bioelectromagnetics Association[72] also document beneficial clinical effects of electromagnetic therapy for patients with multiple sclerosis.

Currently, very exciting case reports are coming from researchers who are doing FDA clinical trials of a device using very strong (3,000- to 5,000-gauss) direct-current (DC) electromagnetic fields to treat patients with a number of neurological conditions, including multiple sclerosis. Neurologist Dr. Larry Pearce, in a paper presented at the 1999 North American

Academy of Magnetic Therapy meeting, noted improvement in vision, speech, gait, memory, and fatigue in seven multiple sclerosis patients who were undergoing treatment at the Dayspring Medical Center in North Carolina with the Magnetic Molecular Energizing (MME) device, invented by Dr. Dean Bonlie of the Advanced Magnetic Research Institute in Calgary, Canada.[73]

Osteoarthritis

Osteoarthritis is the most common form of arthritis, afflicting nearly 21 million Americans. A degenerative joint disease, in which the cartilage that covers and protects the ends of the bones deteriorates, its primary symptoms are pain and loss of mobility.

Orthopedic surgeon Dr. David Stokesbary of the American branch of the Advanced Magnetic Research Institute in Laguna Niguel, California, reports successful relief of osteoarthritic pain in patients who received electromagnetic treatment with the DC Magnetic Molecular Energizing device. This is the same device used by Pearce to treat patients with multiple sclerosis (discussed in the preceding subsection). Stokesbary notes that osteoarthritic patients have remained pain-free one year after completion of treatment.[74]

A number of AC electromagnetic therapy studies have also shown favorable osteoarthritis results. In 1993, researchers in the Department of Medicine at Danbury Hospital in Connecticut conducted a double-blind, placebo-controlled study of the effect of pulsed electromagnetic fields (PEMF) on twenty-seven patients with osteoarthritis, primarily of the knee. In the treated group, an average improvement of 23 to 61 percent in variables related to pain and functional performance was noted. In contrast, the sham group improvement was 2 to 18 percent.[75]

Another double-blind, placebo-controlled study, conducted at the same institution a year later, examined the effects of PEMF on osteoarthritis of the knee and the cervical spine. This was a much larger study, involving eighty-six knee patients and eighty-one cervical patients. PEMF was again found to have resulted in greater improvement in the treated group compared to the sham group for both knee and cervical conditions. In both the Danbury studies, significant improvement differences in the treated groups were maintained one month following completion of the treatment.[76]

Research conducted at Johns Hopkins University of Medicine in Baltimore in 1995 confirmed the Danbury results. In this multicenter, double-blind, placebo-controlled study, seventy-eight patients with osteoarthritis of the knee were given either pulsed therapy or sham treatment for four weeks. Improvements in pain and function were significantly greater for the treated group than the sham group.[77]

Exciting research on knee osteoarthritis has recently been submitted to the FDA as a component of the application for approval of a new electromagnetic healing device. Under the direction of Dr. Roger Gorman, of the Department of Applied Medical Physics and Neuromagnetics at the West Boca Medical Campus in Boca Raton, Florida, a double-blind, placebo-controlled study of 176 patients was undertaken to evaluate the effectiveness of the Jacobson Resonator. Patients were given either eight sham or eight active treatments with the Jacobson Resonator during a two-week period. Immediately after and two weeks after completion of the therapy, the resonator-treated group reported an average 50 percent reduction in pain, whereas the sham group noted an average 8 percent reduction. Ninety-six percent of those in the treatment group reported some benefit in response to the treatment.[78]

The results of other pioneering osteoarthritis research were presented by Canadian physician, electrical engineer, and pain specialist Dr. Cecil Hershler at the 1999 North American Academy of Magnetic Therapy meeting. At the meeting, Dr. Hershler shared the results of a retrospective outcome study of forty-five osteoarthritis patients he had treated using AC pulsed electromagnetic therapy (10 gauss, less than 20 hertz) in his Vancouver clinic. The pulse signal therapy device he employed in the study has been approved for use in Canada, Mexico, the Middle East, and fourteen European countries.

Hershler's review revealed that immediately after completion of the course of nine one-hour treatments, 60 percent of the patients experienced a reduction in both frequency and intensity of chronic arthritic pain. Six weeks after treatment, the percentage of patients experiencing pain relief had increased to 76 percent, and that percentage was maintained at six months.

One of the most fascinating findings of Hershler's research is that the results improved over time—from 60 to 76 percent. Hershler believes that the treatment reactivates the normal streaming potential (movement of positive ions) lost by damaged cartilage cells. With this activity restored, explained Hershler, the cells are able to grow more cartilage, and pain is reduced. In essence, the therapy jump-starts cellular replication, and then the body continues the process.

In the 160 patients Hershler has treated with the device, for both osteoarthritis and soft-tissue injuries (damage to muscles, ligaments, and tendons), 70 to 80 percent have achieved some degree of improvement in function, including sitting, walking, and sleeping.

In one anecdote of a dramatic healing experience, Hershler recounted the story of a film musical composer who was so debilitated by a herniated vertebral disc pressing on a nerve root that he could not sit, stand, or walk. He had to have a computer rigged above his body so he could work from his bed. After just five treatments, the man was walking four miles. A year later, he continued to be pain-free and was leading a full and active life.[79]

Electromagnetic therapy has also been found to be an effective treatment for other bone conditions, including osteoporosis, osteochondrosis (inflammation), and osteonecrosis (cell death).

In terms of static magnets, Lawrence reports that osteoarthritis is the condition he most frequently treats with such magnets in his clinical practice.[80] He has found them helpful in relieving pain symptoms, as have other clinicians, such as Kamhi.[81]

Parkinson's Disease

As with multiple sclerosis, most of the published research on treating Parkinson's disease with electromagnetic fields comes from Sandyk. His numerous case studies describe the beneficial results achieved in treating Parkinson's patients with picotesla electromagnetic fields. Treated patients experienced improvement in a number of areas, including tremor and other motor symptoms, vision, depression, cognitive symptoms, and visual memory.[82]

Transcranial magnetic stimulation—the same treatment found to relieve severe depression—has also been shown to improve Parkinson's disease symptoms.[83] And Pearce, who reported favorable results in treating multiple sclerosis patients with the MME device (discussed in an earlier subsection), noted that all seven Parkinson's patients undergoing treatment with these strong DC electromagnetic fields had shown improvement in tremor, rigidity, and movement.[84]

Post-Polio Syndrome

A double-blind placebo-controlled pilot study was recently undertaken at Baylor University College of Medicine in Houston to investigate the effect of static magnets on post-polio syndrome pain.

Post-polio patients commonly experience muscular and/or arthritic pain. Fifty patients participated in this pilot study and had either an active bipolar (300- to 500-gauss) or a sham bipolar magnet applied over a trigger point associated with an area of referred pain for a treatment period of forty-five minutes. At the end of the one-time treatment period, 76 percent of the patients treated with an active magnet reported a reduction in pain, in contrast to 19 percent of the patients treated with a sham device.[85]

Rheumatoid Arthritis

Although far less common than osteoarthritis, rheumatoid arthritis can be very debilitating. An inflammatory autoimmune disease, rheumatoid arthritis causes severe and painful swelling of the joints.

One Eastern European study documented the beneficial effects of static magnet therapy for patients with rheumatoid arthritis.

Researchers noted improvement in both clinical symptoms and laboratory values for patients in the early stages of the disease.[86]

In other Eastern European studies, some patients with rheumatoid arthritis have been observed to worsen before they improved. Jerabek and Pawluk advise that if this occurs, treatment should not be interrupted, but the frequency of the treatment should be reduced. In cases in which the condition still does not improve, they recommend that the strength of the magnetic field be decreased.[87]

Positive clinical effects have also been observed in the treatment of rheumatoid arthritis with electromagnetic fields.[88]

Skin Problems

An Eastern European study has shown favorable results in using static magnets in treating microbial eczema. Other Eastern European studies have reported beneficial effects from electromagnetic therapy given to patients with atopic (allergic) eczema and dermatitis.[89]

Clinical observations and personal experiences document the usefulness of static magnets for healing minor as well as more severe skin problems. Dr. Michael Tierra, who has treated thousands of patients with magnets, reports successfully treating skin conditions such as eczema, psoriasis, and shingles by applying the north side of a magnet to the most diseased area.[90] Pawluk reports healing his spider bites within half an hour by immediately putting magnets on them.[91] Jules Klapper, president of the Cutting Edge Catalogue and a longtime user of magnets, reports similar results with mosquito bites and kitchen burns.[92] A friend of mine told me that she had applied a tiny magnet over an about-to-erupt pimple before she went to bed and found the blemish gone in the morning. Soon after, threatened with a similar annoyance, I stuck a magnet over the nasty spot—and in less than an hour, it had disappeared.

Soft-Tissue Injuries

The healing of soft-tissue injuries (strains, sprains, and irritations of muscles, ligaments, and tendons) by magnet therapy has received much media attention recently, as professional athletes extol their value.

Bill Romanowski, a Denver Broncos linebacker, credits magnet therapy with getting him off anti-inflammatories and accelerating the healing of his knee after surgery. Senior PGA golf pro Jim Colbert routinely wears magnets while playing to relieve his lower-back pain. The Miami Dolphins football team has been using static magnets for a couple of years now to relieve pain and speed recovery. And magnet therapy is a well-established practice among horse trainers and veterinarians, who have been using them for years to keep racehorses (and their riders) in peak shape.

Japanese researchers have reported success with static magnet therapy for patients suffering from joint pain and chronic and acute muscle pain. In a double-blind, placebo-controlled study of 222 patients, researchers reported pain reduction after five days in 90 percent of those treated with static magnets. In the placebo group, 14 percent reported improvement in symptoms.[93] The recent American studies on using static magnets for treating the muscle pain of fibromyalgia and post-polio syndrome also provide supportive evidence.

Many patients have received beneficial results for soft-tissue injuries with the MME device, reports Stokesbary. As an example, he cites the case of tennis pro Lindsay Davenport. After seven months of suffering with a painful tennis elbow that was unresponsive to other treatments, Davenport came to the Laguna Niguel facility. After 5½ hours of treatment, she was pain-free and back on the pro circuit. Stokesbary also recounts unexpected healing of unrelated symptoms. A patient, for example, who came for treatment for an autoimmune disease that caused severe skin symptoms completed treatment healed of the skin problems—and of tennis elbow.[94]

Scientists have also shown AC electromagnetic treatment to be effective in treating soft-tissue problems. In a recent Spanish study, researchers investigated the use of repetitive electromagnetic stimulation on localized musculoskeletal pain. In the placebo-controlled study, thirty patients were randomly assigned to receive forty minutes of real or sham treatment. After a single session, the pain scores of the magnetically treated group dropped 59 percent, whereas those who received the sham treatment reported a decrease of 14 percent. The pain relief was sustained for several days after the treatment.[95]

In another recent double-blind, placebo-controlled study, researchers investigated the effect of pulsed radio-frequency therapy on the healing of ankle sprains. They found that two thirty-minute sessions significantly speeded the reduction of edema.[96]

In a study published in *Lancet*, researchers described the favorable results of pulsed electromagnetic therapy on patients suffering from long-standing tendinitis of the rotator cuff. At the end of the sixteen-week study, nineteen (65 percent) of the twenty-nine treated patients were symptomless, and another five patients were much improved.[97]

Irish researchers have investigated the effect of pulsed electromagnetic therapy on acute whiplash. In a double-blind, placebo-controlled study of forty patients, those who received active therapy collars had significantly less pain and improved range of motion in comparison to those who wore placebo collars.[98]

Remember the exciting pain reduction effects reported by Hershler for osteoarthritis patients he treated with pulsed electromagnetic therapy? He also found that the same beneficial effects occurred in patients suffering with soft-tissue problems.

Yet more evidence comes from the many bone-fracture studies performed by Eastern European researchers. Employing either static or electromagnetic fields, the scientists repeatedly noted that the therapy resulted in accelerated healing not only of the fractures but also of soft tissues. Beneficial effects included prevention or reduction of edema and decreased pain and tissue inflammation.[99]

Recovery from Surgery

In one reported Eastern European study, 138 patients were treated with static magnet therapy immediately after undergoing spinal surgery. In the majority of treated patients, marked analgesia was noted within three to four days. Compared to the untreated control group, healing was faster, edema was markedly reduced, and sutures were removed two to three days earlier.[100]

In another Eastern European study, 245 patients were treated with static magnet therapy prior to undergoing phlebectomy (surgical removal of a vein). The magnetically treated patients, according to researchers, healed twelve to twenty days faster than those who did not receive treatment.[101]

Other Eastern European researchers have reviewed the results of twenty years of experience using static magnets in the treatment of more than four thousand gynecological surgery patients. Positive results observed included analgesia, edema reduction, and stimulation of healing.[102]

American researchers, led by Dr. Daniel Man, recently conducted an observational study of the effect of static magnet therapy on twenty-one liposuction surgery patients at a plastic and laser surgery center in Boca Raton, Florida. After the liposuction procedure, magnetic pads were placed over the patients' operative region and left in place for 48 hours. The treated areas were inspected 24, 36, 48, and 72 hours after placement. In approximately 60 percent of the patients, pain, edema, and discoloration were diminished. The symptoms disappeared completely in 75 percent of those who responded to magnet therapy.[103] Man claims similar results for patients who have undergone reconstructive and other plastic surgery procedures at his center and believes that recovery time is usually decreased 50 percent or more by postsurgical magnet application.

Electromagnetic therapy has also been found to speed recovery after surgery. Eastern European researchers have reported success with electromagnetic therapy in gynecologic surgery. When six hundred patients with endometriosis were treated before and immediately after surgery, wound healing was accelerated, and there was an absence of complications in the postoperative period.[104]

Wound Healing

A number of Eastern European studies attest to the effectiveness of static magnets in healing wounds and burns. In one study, in which researchers used static magnets to treat twenty-nine patients with gunshot or explosion wounds, it was found that microcirculation was improved, edema was reduced, and healing of soft tissue was accelerated.[105]

In a controlled study of seventy-five patients with first- to third-degree burns on less than 10 percent of their body surface, the application of static magnets resulted in pain relief after the second exposure. Regrowth of skin started within seven to nine days in treated patients. In contrast, skin regrowth in the control group began on day fourteen.[106]

Another group of researchers compared both static and electromagnetic therapy in the same population—patients with first- to third-degree burns on less than 10 percent of their body surface. In this study of forty-six patients, it was found that those who received static magnet treatment had normalized histamine levels on the fourth day, whereas the histamine levels of those who received electromagnetic treatment normalized on the fourteenth day. The researchers concluded that static field therapy was better.[107]

Here in the United States, a case study was published in 1998 describing the use of static magnet therapy to heal an abdominal wound. The researchers, from Toledo Hospital in Toledo, Ohio, describe the treatment of a fifty-one-year-old paraplegic woman with an abdominal wound that had been resistant to conventional approaches for a year. After a magnet was placed over her abdominal dressing for one month, the wound completely healed.[108]

A report from the Institute for Biophysics and Ray-Research in Vienna, Austria, provides evidence that the application of static magnets can result in the amelioration of scars. Treatment with bipolar magnetic strips (foils) of patients with postoperative and burn scars resulted in pain relief and, after approximately four to five months, disintegration of scars.[109]

There have also been numerous published studies regarding the effectiveness of electromagnetic therapy in healing a variety of wounds, including venous leg ulcers and nonhealing amputation stumps.

Other Studies

Given the scope of this book and its focus on static magnets, a comprehensive review of the electromagnetic literature was not possible. In addition to the conditions reviewed in this chapter, you can find published electromagnetic studies for a wide variety of other ailments, including Alzheimer's disease, amyotrophic lateral sclerosis (Lou Gehrig's disease), glaucoma, hemophilia, hepatitis, intestinal ulcers, kidney and urinary problems, lupus erythematosus, male-pattern baldness, nerve damage, otitis externa, pancreatitis, spinal cord injury, sexual disorders, stroke, throat and respiratory conditions, and tuberculosis.

Although studies have been published in which electromagnetic treatment combined with conventional therapy was shown to be beneficial in the treatment of cancer, very little is known yet about the effect of static magnets. Experts advise against self-treatment until more research has been completed.

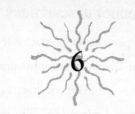

Choosing Magnets

WANDERING THE MAGNETIC WEB

When you enter *magnet therapy* into your computer's Web browser, you'll probably get about fifteen hundred listings. Most of those entries belong to distributors promoting a wide variety of biomagnetic products.

Just browsing magnet therapy Web sites and catalogs can be daunting. Frankly, I was quite overwhelmed as I cruised through competitor catalogs and advertisements. There were so many different varieties and types. And some of the terminology used to describe the products might as well have been in Greek, for as much sense as it originally made to me.

Hopefully, I can now dispel some of the confusion for you—and provide some practical guidelines for evaluating and purchasing biomagnetic products.

PRODUCT DESCRIPTIONS

Static (also known as permanent or stationary) biomagnets are frequently described or labeled as "nonmedical devices." One of the larger manufacturers of magnetic devices says its products are to be used for "rest and relaxation." The reason for such language is that the Food and Drug Administration (FDA) has not approved static magnets as medical devices. Some manufacturers that have made medical claims have had their inventory seized and their doors permanently shuttered. So until there is sufficient research to win FDA approval of static magnets as medical devices, we will continue to see such descriptions.

TYPES OF MAGNETIC PRODUCTS

Today, a wide variety of static magnet products is available in the marketplace. Some can be found in chain drug and department stores. Others can only be ordered from catalogs or sales representatives. Let's look at the most common types.

- *Individual magnets:* Healing magnets come in a variety of sizes and shapes to fit various body areas. Popular sizes for treating small areas include half-inch to inch disks and credit-card-size rectangles. Larger square and rectangular forms are designed to be applied to areas like the back and shoulders. Some are made of Plastiform—a flexible plastic material. Designed for hard-to-reach spots, they can be cut into a variety of shapes. Individual magnets are commonly held in place by adhesive tape, pads, or wraps. Some companies sell an assortment pack of various sizes and shapes—a magnetic first-aid kit.

- *Point magnets:* These are tiny magnets attached to the sticky side of a round adhesive bandage. The bandages are usually about half an inch in diameter and look like the little circular Band-Aids you apply to tiny boo-boos. These devices are used on acupuncture points (see chapter 7) and can be handy for about-to-erupt pimples or other small, minor skin irritations.

- *Block magnets:* Block magnets commonly come in a 4-inch by 6-inch size, with a half-inch depth. They are designed to be placed under mattresses, pillows, and seat cushions or propped against a headboard. They are also the type recommended for magnetizing a container of water.

- *Body wraps:* Body wraps are made of elasticized or other flexible material and are usually secured by a Velcro closure. Some products have the magnets enclosed in the wrap, whereas others contain slots or other openings, which allow the magnets to be inserted and removed at will. Some wraps can be used for a variety of body ᵣ whereas others are specifically designed fo⸱ ⸱ ankle, elbow, shoulder, wrist, hand, nᵢ

Healing Magnets

- *Mattresses and mattress pads:* You have a choice between mattresses embedded with magnets or thinner magnetic mattress pads, designed to be placed either on top of your existing mattress or between your box spring and mattress.

- *Pillows:* Pillows with embedded magnets, some ergonomically designed, are available to complement your magnetic mattress.

- *Seats:* These products are designed to provide magnetic therapy to your back and bottom. Portable, they can easily be moved from home to car to office and back again.

- *Insoles:* Magnetic insoles slip inside your shoes. They typically come in one size, which you cut to fit your shoes. There is variety in thickness and the flexibility of the material used.

- *Massage devices:* Both static and battery-powered magnetic massagers are offered by some manufacturers.

- *Jewelry:* A variety of jewelry products is available. The most commonly seen are necklaces, pendants, and bracelets. In design, they range from earthy to high-tech to high-fashion. Take your pick.

- *Clothing:* Magnetic vests and belts can now be purchased. Who knows what's coming next?

- *Beauty products:* Some manufacturers offer magnetic face masks. (Cleopatra would've loved this one!) Some are designed with embedded magnets, claiming to fall over acupuncture points or the most common wrinkle lines. Others allow the user to individually position the magnets.

A variety of other beauty-oriented products are beginning to appear on the market. A cosmetics manufacturer has developed skin products that incorporate micromagnetic particles. Increasing blood circulation leads to enhanced glow, claims the company. I've gotten word of magnetized combs to attract dandruff. If they're not already in the pipeline, I'm sure magnetic toothpaste and oral irrigators are coming soon.

- *Water treatment:* Magnetic water conditioners come in a variety of forms that can be attached to the incoming water line in your home, to the output from a water heater, and to faucets and showerheads.

- *Animal products:* Based on the successful experience of trainers and veterinarians with racehorses, manufacturers are offering not only equine magnetic blankets but also blankets for smaller animals (dogs and cats) and pet-size sleeping pads.

PURCHASING CONSIDERATIONS

When thinking about purchasing a magnetic product, you should consider a number of factors.

Strength

The jury is still very much out on how strong is strong enough to achieve an effect. There haven't yet been enough studies to let us know what is optimal magnetic field strength.

As you may recall from chapter 3, magnet strength is most commonly described in units called gauss, which are measured by sensitive, calibrated instruments called gaussmeters. Gauss is actually a measure of the density of magnetic flux lines. The more magnetic flux lines per square centimeter, the higher the gauss number—and the more powerful the magnet.

GAUSS RATINGS

There are two types of gauss ratings: internal and external. Manufacturers measure and assign a manufacturer gauss rating, which tells you the internal strength of the magnet. The other type of rating is called a surface gauss rating, which tells you the magnetic strength at the external surface of the magnet. There can be quite a difference between the two ratings. For example, one neodymium product I examined had a 12,000-gauss manufacturer rating and a 1,000- to 1,500-gauss surface rating.

Scientists, therapists, and manufacturers note that the surface strength of a magnet depends on a number of factors, including the size and shape of the product, the type and grade of the magnetic material, and the polarity orientation. One magnet therapist who measured a number of products of the same man-

ufacturer gauss strength with a gaussmeter found a wide varia-
tion in their surface ratings.[1] *In any case, it is the surface rating, not the*
manufacturer rating, to which we should pay attention—and that we should
use to compare products.

The surface rating, however, doesn't give us the whole story
because magnetic fields fall off exponentially, equal to the
square of the distance from the surface of the magnet. Given
this fact, you wouldn't need as strong a magnet to treat a burn at
the surface of the skin as you would to treat a muscle 1 to 2
inches beneath the skin. Table 6-1 gives you an idea of what this
looks like in terms of actual measurements.

TABLE 6-1
Magnetic Strength (Actual Measurements)

Surface	436 gauss
1 inch	268 gauss
2 inches	161 gauss
4 inches	63 gauss
8 inches	27 gauss

Source: Results of an informal experiment conducted by Dr. John Zimmerman, September 18,
1999, using a gaussmeter to measure magnetic field strength both at the center of the surface of a
ceramic magnet and at various distances from the surface.

OPTIMAL STRENGTH

So what do the experts say about optimal magnetic field strength? Dr. John Zimmerman notes that anecdotal evidence suggests that the stronger the magnet, the quicker the pain relief. Dr. Michael Tierra, who has treated thousands of patients for pain and inflammation with magnets, regularly uses no less than 3,000 gauss. Physicist Dr. Marko Markov suggests that 400 to 500 gauss is an optimal strength *at the tissue level*. Depending on how deep the area you are treating, you would need to use magnets with very high surface gauss ratings.

A number of magnet therapists have noted that treatment is more effective when magnets are placed over acupuncture points. Acupuncturists who use tiny point magnets on acupuncture points have found 500 to 600 gauss to be very effective. And the strength of the static magnets used in the Eastern European studies reviewed by Drs. Jiri Jerabek and William Pawluk ranged from 100 to 500 gauss.

In terms of safety, the World Health Organization (WHO) concluded in 1987 that "available knowledge indicates the absence of any adverse effects on human health due to exposure to static magnet fields up to 2 tesla (20,000 gauss)."[2]

Material

Biomagnetic products are made of different magnetic materials. The most common are ferrites, a type of ceramic material, composed of iron oxides combined with cobalt, nickel, barium, or other metals. Many manufacturers use the terms *ferrite* and *ceramic* interchangeably.

To make flexible magnets that can easily wrap around a body part or fit in odd-shaped nooks and crannies, manufacturers combine a ferrite mixture with plastic, rubber, or other pliable material. These products tend to be weaker in strength than magnets composed solely of ferrite or ceramic.

You will also see neodymium magnets advertised. These products are actually an alloy of the rare earth element neodymium combined with iron and boron. This material is able to hold more magnetism and is currently the strongest permanent biomagnet available.

Unipolar versus Bipolar

Magnet products are available in both unipolar and bipolar forms. Whether bipolar or unipolar magnets are more effective is one of the most controversial topics today among magnet researchers and therapists.

As you may recall from chapter 4, a unipolar magnet product is one in which only one pole or a series of the same pole (either north *or* south but not both) faces the body, while the opposite pole faces away from the body. Some scientists call them unidirectional magnets. Informational material included with unipolar magnets usually tells you which side of the product is the north (negative) side.

In contrast, bipolar magnetic products are designed in such a way that *both* poles (north *and* south) face the body. Bipolar products are designed in a variety of alternating spatial patterns. The most common are concentric circles, checkerboard, stripes, and triangles. Each manufacturer claims that its pattern is the best, and some have credible studies showing that its magnets are effective compared to placebo treatment. Until we have comparative studies of all patterns, we won't know whether they actually vary in effectiveness.

Some manufacturers use unipolar magnets in some products and bipolar in others, and many magnet distributors sell both types. Deciding whether to purchase a unipolar or bipolar product depends on the school of thought to which you adhere. See chapter 7 for more on this topic.

Uniformity of Field

As scientists like Markov, Pawluk, and Zimmerman explain, although magnetic products with all same-pole magnets facing one direction are called unipolar, technically a complete unipolar field doesn't exist. If you take a magnetometer and measure the field of the north side of a magnet, the instrument will read north until just beyond the very edges. At that point, it will read south. Likewise, if you measure the field of the south side of a magnet, it will be south until just beyond the edges. Then, it will switch to north. This phenomenon is called "opposite-pole bleed-through."

If you believe that the north (negative) side of the magnet is the preferred healing side, you will want to avoid any south pole bleed-through. The way to eliminate or reduce this effect is to use a magnet that is larger than the area you are treating. For mattresses and pads, Zimmerman advises that a unipolar field can be attained "by employing a larger number of magnets, spaced closer together, and employing a spacer pad of some thickness between the magnets and the user."[3] The more magnets used, the heavier and more expensive the product becomes, but if you want a pure negative field, this is a factor you may want to consider.

Money-Back Guarantee

Even though manufacturers and distributors legally can't promise results, if the company offers a thirty-day money-back guarantee, this gives you some assurance that the company takes pride in its products and is willing to stand behind them. A listing of magnet distributors is included in appendix I.

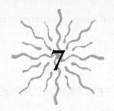

7

Treating with Magnets

PROFESSIONAL INTEREST

A variety of health-care professionals—physicians, naturopaths, acupuncturists, chiropractors, massage therapists, and so forth—have incorporated static magnet therapy into their practice in the last few years. Although many are known only by word of mouth, there are a few resources, listed in appendix I, that may help you find a magnet therapist in your area. With new professional training programs emerging, their number should be growing.

When you hear the stories of professionals (and many researchers) who have gotten involved with magnet therapy, the propelling factor was frequently patients, staff, friends, or relatives who had benefited from self-treatment. Although consulting an experienced practitioner, who has seen hundreds or thousands of patients, may be a wise move for more complicated problems, magnet therapy, in most cases, is something you can safely pursue on your own.

A FEW PRECAUTIONS

All of the clinicians with whom I consulted cautioned that you should see a physician if you have acute or persistent *undiagnosed pain*. Such pain may indicate a serious problem that requires more than magnet therapy.

Otherwise, given what we know and don't know about static magnets, most experts believe that self-therapy is safe, except in the following situations:

- Pregnancy
- Bleeding wounds
- Internal bleeding
- Blood thinner usage (such as Coumadin)
- Epilepsy
- Implanted devices (pacemakers, insulin pumps, and so on)
- Implanted metal plates, screws, and so forth (avoid the area)
- Immediately after eating (wait sixty to ninety minutes)

In addition, Drs. Jiri Jerabek and William Pawluk caution against using magnet therapy if you have clinically symptomatic endocrine dysfunction (thyroid, adrenals, and so forth), myasthenia gravis, active tuberculosis, acute viral diseases, cancer, or psychoses.[1]

Dr. Xiu Ling Ma notes that Chinese researchers have documented that magnet therapy can decrease the white blood cell count (WBC) in patients who already have a below-normal level. If you tend to get one infection after another, it would be wise to get your WBC measured before you engage in magnet therapy.[2] Ma, like other traditional Oriental medicine (TOM) practitioners I consulted, advises against the use of magnets if you are very debilitated.

There's one more precaution to take—and this one is nonmedical. Healing magnets are very strong and can affect watches and erase magnetically stored information on video- and audiotapes, computer disks, CDs, and magnetized cards (credit, debit, and so forth). Be sure to keep magnets several inches from these items.

A COMPLEMENTARY THERAPY

Magnet therapy is not a magic bullet. But enough evidence has been accumulated to support its use for pain relief and for speeding recovery from sports injuries and other traumas. It may also offer more subtle and long-lasting benefits—by restoring balance to our organs and cells.

Magnet therapy works by itself and also synergistically with other nontoxic therapies. Particularly when the goal is reduction of inflammation and the associated pain, magnet therapists have found that adding anti-inflammatory natural remedies can bring quicker relief.

Neurologist Dr. Ron Lawrence has found this to be true with methyl-sulfonyl-methane (MSM), a natural organic sulfur, derived from pine trees.[3] Depending on the nature of the inflammatory condition, Dr. Ellen Kahmi's recommendations may include glucosamine sulfate, black radish, ginger, white willow bark, licorice root, feverfew, and kava kava.[4] Swiss naturopath Dr. Holger Hannemann recommends adding homeopathic remedies, along with good nutrition, massage, hydrotherapy, and exercise.[5]

Massage and chiropractic therapy are good complements to magnets, as they both assist in restoring the body's natural balance. And placing magnets over acupuncture points has been found to be very effective (see the "Acupuncture Points" subsection later in the chapter).

THE POLARITY ISSUE

As I noted in the last chapter, some magnet therapists believe that bipolar magnets are more effective, whereas others maintain that unipolar magnets are the way to go.

Those who support the bipolar view, like Pawluk, cite evidence such as the positive results of the many Eastern European studies in which the researchers used chessboard-pattern bipolar magnets to heal a variety of conditions.

The idea that the north and south poles of a magnet produce different effects originated with the 1930s research of Dr.

Albert Roy Davis and Walter C. Rawls Jr. Dr. William Philpott claims to have validated their ideas through his clinical practice and observations over the last couple of decades. His description of some of the effects of north (negative) and south (positive) magnetic energy is summarized in table 7-1.

TABLE 7-I
Unique Properties of North and South Pole Energy

North (Negative) Pole Energy	South (Positive) Pole Energy
Relieves/stops pain	Increases pain
Reduces inflammation	Can increase inflammation
Normalizes acid-base balance	Promotes an acidic metabolic response
Supports biological healing	Inhibits biological healing
Reduces fluid retention	Increases fluid retention
Fights infection	Accelerates microorganism growth
Facilitates deep, restorative sleep	Stimulates wakefulness

Source: W. Philpott and S. L. Taplin, *Biomagnetic Handbook: Today's Introduction to the Energy Medicine of Tomorrow* (Choctaw, Okla.: Enviro-Tech Products, 1990), 6.

Some magnet therapists have validated Philpott's findings in their clinical practices, and many consumers have received healing benefits from the application of a north pole magnetic field. In terms of popular usage right now, the north pole is generally considered the "healing" side. Most manufacturers identify the north side of their products so you can easily tell which side you should use.

There are a few other viewpoints, however, that should be mentioned. Dr. Buryl Payne, who has been researching magnetic healing for many years, feels that the south pole is generally more healing. He bases his conclusions on his clinical experience and observations of plant growth.[6]

Tom Nellessen, who has been involved with magnet therapy for nearly thirty years, maintains that both poles have specific healing abilities. According to Nellessen, the north pole slows down electrons, whereas the south pole accelerates them. In treating a condition such as tennis elbow, Nellessen would use the north side first to decrease the inflammation and then use the south side to strengthen the joint.[7]

Physicist Dr. Marko Markov believes that both unipolar and bipolar magnets have their place as healing tools. In describing the physics of bipolar and unipolar magnets, Markov explains that bipolar magnets have a limited depth of penetration—.6 to .8 inch. His position is that bipolar magnets are suitable for superficial applications but that unipolar magnets, which have a greater depth of penetration, should be used to treat areas more distant from the body's surface. Because there is no controlled published research validating that either the north or south pole is more effective, Markov thinks it doesn't make any difference which pole of a unipolar magnet you use.[8]

HOW TO USE MAGNETS

Bandage Approach

The most commonly used method of magnet therapy is simply to position the magnet over the area to be treated.

- Place the magnet as close to the surface of your skin as possible, since the strength of the magnet decreases so dramatically with distance.

- If you want a stronger field, stack one magnet on top of another. Magnetic force is accumulative.

- If your problem involves a joint (wrist, ankle, knee, and so forth), some therapists recommend surrounding the entire joint.

- Wraps or adhesive tape are the easiest ways to hold magnets in place.

For Unipolar Magnets

A few additional considerations need to be taken into account when using a unipolar magnet:

- If you are using the north side to relieve pain and it gets worse, flip to the other side. Sometimes the manufacturer incorrectly identifies polarity. And as you learned in the preceding section, some magnet therapists think the south side is more effective.

- To prevent opposite-pole bleed-through, choose a magnet with dimensions larger than the area you are treating.

- According to Philpott, the north side pulls fluid. If you are treating an enclosed swollen area, such as sinuses or joints, Philpott recommends that you place the magnet a little distance away from the affected area to drain the fluid and relieve the pressure. For application of this principle to headaches, see chapter 5.

Points, Points, and More Points

The other approach to using magnets is to place them over specific identified points on the body's surface.

TRIGGER POINTS

You may recall that the successful treatment of pain in post-polio patients, described in chapter 5, involved placing the magnets on trigger points. Trigger points are most often found in skeletal muscles and their tendons. Touching these sensitive points can cause pain locally—or in a distant location (referred pain), such as is often the case with the post-polio patients.

Trigger points have been found, like acupuncture points, to have increased electrical activity. Interestingly, it has been discovered that there is a 71 percent correspondence between both the spatial distribution and the associated pain pathways of traditional acupuncture points and trigger points.[9]

TREATING TRIGGER POINTS

If your pain has not been relieved with the application of a magnet to the local area, you might try to discover an associated trigger point. If you have pain, for example, in your upper arm, palpate up toward your shoulder and down below your elbow. You'll know a trigger point when you find one. It can be very tender to the touch, and you will feel the pain travel from the identified "ouch" point to the area you have been treating. Once that point has been found, place a magnet over it. Some magnet therapists, like Lawrence, think it's best to treat both the local and referred areas at the same time.

ACUPUNCTURE POINTS

Traditional Oriental medicine (TOM) views the human organism as a dynamic energy system. According to the TOM model, the body has fourteen major energy pathways, called meridians, through which the body's vital force (*chi* or *qi*) flows. Each pathway is associated with particular body organs and physical and psychological functions. The liver meridian, for example, is associated not only with the liver but also with the muscles, tendons, nails, eyes, reproductive system, the emotion of anger, and the ability to plan. Optimal health is attained when energy flows unimpeded through all the meridians.

Located along each meridian are specific points that are bioelectrically charged. Acupuncture—the stimulation of these points by hair-thin needles—activates the body's energy. Classical theory recognizes about 365 points on the major meridians. However, when you add the lesser meridians, ear points, and other miscellaneous points that have been identified, the total number of bioelectrically sensitive points increases to 2,000.[10]

Acupuncture has been one of the primary healing tools of TOM for more than four thousand years. After being introduced into the United States in the early 1970s, its popularity as a healing modality has steadily increased. In 1997, acupuncture was acknowledged by the National Institutes of Health's Consensus Development Panel as a useful treatment for a variety of painful conditions, including headaches, menstrual cramps, osteoarthritis, low-back pain, and carpal tunnel syndrome.[11]

Although manual needling is the best known form of point stimulation, other methods are also used, including electrical needle stimulation, finger pressure (acupressure), lasers, and moxibustion—the application of heat from burning mugwort (moxa). Some TOM practitioners in the United States have followed the lead of their Asian counterparts in using tiny magnets for point stimulation.

TREATING ACUPUNCTURE POINTS

Pioneers in magnet therapy, such as Lawrence and Pawluk, discovered that magnet therapy could be very effective when the magnets were placed over acupuncture points.

There are two ways to go about this. You can be very precise and place a tiny point magnet over an identified acupuncture point. Or if you are using a larger magnet, you will end up placing the magnet over the point and the surrounding area. Favorable results have been reported with both approaches.

Some points that are helpful for some common conditions are included in appendix 2. Using the illustrations and point location descriptions as guides, feel around until you find an "ouch" spot. When the energy is congested in a point, it will usually be tender. For more information on points that are useful for self-treatment, see a more extensive source, such as Michael Reed Gach's *Acupressure's Potent Points: A Guide to Self-Care for Common Ailments.*[12]

Incidentally, even if you aren't intentionally treating an acupuncture point, any surface magnet will probably be contacting one or more points, since there are so many of them. For example, if you put a magnet-containing wrap around your wrist, you'll probably be contacting Pericardium 6 and 7 (P 6 and 7) as well as Triple Warmer 4 and 5 (TW 4 and 5).

Healing Magnets

KOREAN HAND POINTS

Korean Hand Therapy (KHT) is practiced by 50,000 health-care practitioners in Korea. Some 4 to 5 million Koreans use the system for self-treatment. It is so popular in Brazil that a Korean Hand Therapy holiday is celebrated each year in São Paulo. Here in the United States, KHT has been gaining popularity during the last decade, as a growing number of acupuncturists, chiropractors, massage therapists, and everyday people attend training workshops.

Developed in 1971 by Dr. Tae-Woo Yoo, a well-respected South Korean TOM practitioner, KHT maps out the entire human body and major internal organs as well as a whole system of micromeridians on each hand that, with a few exceptions, correspond to the TOM body meridians.

According to Yoo, there are more somatic nerve connections between the hand and the brain than any other body part, and this is one of the underlying reasons this healing system has such good results. Several well-seasoned acupuncturists (ten to fifteen years in practice) with whom I spoke at a training work-shop now use KHT as their primary mode of treatment. They have found it clinically to be much more effective than treating traditional body points.

Although more complicated problems may need the assistance of a KHT-trained practitioner, many conditions can be treated on your own. Various means are used to stimulate the hand points, including tiny needles, silver- and gold-colored metal pellets, moxa, electrical stimulation—and magnets.

TREATING KOREAN HAND POINTS

In general, problems on the front side of the body are treated on the palm side of the hand, whereas problems on the back part of the body are treated on the top side of the hand. Problems with the right limbs are primarily treated on the right ring and little fingers, whereas the left limbs are primarily treated on the left ring and little fingers. Problems in the center of the body are treated on the micromeridian that runs from the tip of the middle finger to the wrist. (See appendix 3.)

Treatment points are identified by probing with a sharp object to find one or more "ouch" points (distinctly more painful than other probed areas), and then 600-gauss point magnets are applied. Because the treatment is so powerful, KHT practitioners advise leaving the magnets in place no longer than twenty to forty minutes.

Detailed instructional materials, point magnets and other supplies, and workshop schedules are available from KHT Systems (see appendix I).

More Generalized Treatment

Sleeping on magnetic mattresses, sitting on magnetic pads, and wearing magnetic jewelry and insoles have all been promoted as ways to achieve whole-body treatment. There are currently no guidelines other than manufacturer instructions about these products. You just need to experiment and find out what works or doesn't work for you.

Drinking magnetic water has also been promoted by some magnet therapists as a way to enhance overall energy and wellness. As with most other areas of magnetic therapy, there is quite a diversity of opinion about how to magnetize water. Presented in tables 7-2 and 7-3 are the very different recommendations of two magnet therapists—Philpott and Hannemann.

FREQUENTLY ASKED QUESTIONS

- *Will I feel anything?* Some people have a sensation of heat, tingling, or itching when they use magnets. Others feel nothing at all. Remember, if you are using a unipolar magnet and your pain increases, try the other side.

- *How long should I leave the magnets on?* Here again, as in other areas of magnet therapy, there are different opinions. Some practitioners advise that you treat continuously until your condition is resolved. Others think you should treat intermittently, particularly when using whole-body treatment like magnetic mattresses for long-standing problems, such as chronic fatigue or fibromyalgia.

  Those who propose intermittent treatment are concerned that the body will become used (habituated) to the

TABLE 7-2

Philpott's Magnetic Water Instructions

***

For a Calming Effect

1. Place water in glass container.
2. Set filled container on negative pole of a magnet or tape magnets to container with negative pole directed toward contents.
3. Treat for a minimum of five minutes, preferably longer.
4. Drink a minimum of two 8-ounce glasses daily. During flu epidemic, drink magnetically treated water every four hours for prevention or relief of symptoms.

For Quicker Energy Pick-up in Morning

1. Place water in glass container.
2. Place negative pole of a magnet on one side of filled container and positive magnetic pole on the opposite side.
3. Treat water for a minimum of five minutes before drinking.
4. Drink one 8-ounce glass.

Source: W. Philpott and S. L. Taplin, *Biomagnetic Handbook: Today's Introduction to the Energy Medicine of Tomorrow* (Choctaw, Okla.: Enviro-Tech Products, 1990), 30.

TABLE 7-3

Hannemann's Magnetic Water Instructions

For Activating, Cleansing, and Detoxifying the System

1. Place one or more magnets (total of 2,000 gauss) with south pole pointing up under a container of water at night.
2. Leave the magnet(s) under the container for ten hours.
3. Drink half a glass of the water on an empty stomach first thing in the morning.
4. Drink a total of 1 liter a day, divided into four equal portions.
5. Do not refrigerate the water.
6. Continue the water therapy over several months.

Source: H. Hannemann, *Magnet Therapy: Balancing Your Body's Energy Flow for Self-Healing* (New York: Sterling Publishing, 1990), 32.

---

applied magnetic field and adjust to it. As a result, its healing effects will be diminished. This is the same reason many holistic practitioners advise that you periodically take a break from natural supplements or switch brands.

- *Is there a window of opportunity for certain conditions?* In terms of an acute soft-tissue injury, such as a strained or sprained muscle, immediate application has been found to be very effective in bringing down swelling and enhancing the healing process. Immediate application has also been found to work well for minor skin irritations such as pimples, insect bites, and kitchen burns.

- *Can I overtreat?* Magnets are very powerful, particularly when they are placed over acupuncture points—either intentionally or unintentionally. This is why KHT practitioners advise leaving the magnets on no longer than forty minutes. Pawluk reports putting a couple of magnets on his face at bedtime to treat a sinus problem and then waking up in the middle of the night with an intense buzzing sensation up and down his chest. When he removed the magnets, the sensation stopped. He realized later that the stimulation of the acupuncture points under the magnets had activated one of the major meridians.

- *Is magnet therapy safe?* Because there is evidence that prolonged exposure to extremely low frequency (ELF) electromagnetic fields is associated with cancer and glandular imbalances, there are some concerns that excessive electromagnetic treatment might cause damage. Jerabek and Pawluk, for example, recommend that electromagnetic treatment be limited to no more than one hour per day.[13] Static magnets, on the other hand, are considered safe up to 20,000 gauss. The worst thing that can happen is that you may have some type of reaction, such as Pawluk did, if a meridian is overstimulated. The solution is quite simple. If you feel anything unusual happening in your body, just remove the magnets.

- *Will magnet therapy work for me?* Magnet therapy has benefited many people worldwide. Since everyone is unique, no one can predict whether static magnet therapy will work for you or your particular problem. How strong is strong enough, how long is long enough, and what works for different conditions are today's hottest research questions. But given that magnets are safe, reusable, and inexpensive—compared to most pharmaceuticals—they certainly are worth a try.

For pain relief, magnets are a nontoxic alternative to damaging acetaminophen (Tylenol) and nonsteroidal anti-inflammatory drugs (NSAIDs), like ibuprofen (Advil, Aleve, Motrin) and aspirin. Many people have been able to reduce or eliminate such pain medications. You can speed the healing of acute injuries and potentially avoid long-term immobilization or surgery. And if you do need surgery, magnet therapy can speed your recovery. For everyday minor maladies—like mosquito bites, skin eruptions, and kitchen burns—they can offer almost immediate healing.

The bottom line? Magnets are potent, safe, reusable healing tools. Adding them to your natural medicine chest just makes good sense.

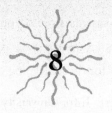

8

Around the Corner

LEARNING MORE

When I asked the experts, "What is the most important issue in static magnet therapy?" they invariably replied, "We need more research." And just as this book was going to press, I attended the 2000 meeting of the North American Academy of Magnetic Therapy, where some new and exciting findings were presented on both static magnets and electromagnetic therapy. Here are a few highlights from the conference:

- *Fibromyalgia* (Taylor, University of Virginia, Center for the Study of Complementary and Alternative Therapies). Patients who slept on magnetic mattresses for six months (in addition to undergoing conventional treatment) showed an improvement in symptoms compared to those who slept on sham mattresses or who received only conventional therapy. The decrease in pain or improvement in functional ability was greater for patients sleeping on north unipolar mattresses than bipolar mattresses, although tender point relief was greater for those sleeping on bipolar mattresses.[1]

- *Depression* (Colbert, Tufts University School of Medicine, Department of Physical Medicine and Rehabilitation). Wearing a baseball cap fitted with magnets, which touched selected acupuncture points on the top of the head, improved symptoms in patients with mild to moderate depression. Seventy percent of the patients who wore the caps twenty to sixty minutes daily during the six-week period experienced some relief.[2]

- *Heart disease* (Stokesbary, Advanced Magnetic Research Institute, Laguna Niguel, California). Post-stroke and congestive heart failure symptoms were significantly improved by the application of very strong direct-current electromagnetic fields, using the Magnetic Molecular Energizing (MME) device.

- *Chronic low back pain* (Zimmerman, Veterans Administration Medical Center, Prescott, Arizona). No difference in pain relief from spondylosis (disk degeneration) was found between those patients who wore bipolar magnets and those who wore placebos for 18 hours. The next trial will evaluate the effects of north unipolar magnets under the same experimental conditions.[3]

- *Recovery from surgery* (Hottentot, Pine Tree Orthopedics, Waterville, Maine). Decreased pain and accelerated healing were achieved with the application of bipolar magnets to orthopedic patients after surgery. A 93 percent satisfaction rate in more than eleven hundred orthopedic patients treated with bipolar magnets was reported.[4]

- *Bone healing* (Rogachefsky, Long Island, New York). The nonhealing wrist (scaphoid) fractures of those patients who had a unipolar north magnet applied to the skin after surgery healed in five weeks, whereas the fractures in the placebo group took eight weeks to heal.[5]

- *Cancer* (Markov, EMF Therapeutics, Inc., Chattanooga, Tennessee). In controlled experiments with mice, the application of a pulsed electromagnetic field resulted in the reduction of the growth of new blood vessels (angiogenesis) in induced cancerous tumors. As angiogenesis is a factor in many diseases, including cancer, macular degeneration, diabetic neuropathy, and multiple sclerosis, this therapy offers great potential promise. Human trials are currently underway.[6]

NERVE REGENERATION

One of the most exciting areas of magnet therapy research is nerve regeneration. Dr. Betty Sisken, University of Kentucky neurobiologist and president of the Bioelectromagnetics

115

Society, has been investigating the effect of both pulsed electromagnetic fields and static magnetic fields on peripheral (other than the brain and spinal cord) nerve growth in chick embryos. She has found that when growth factor is added to the cells, both electromagnetic and static fields increase nerve growth. Although her initial work with static magnets found no difference in results between application of a north pole and a south pole, she is continuing her investigations in this area.[7]

Other pioneering work using picotesla electromagnetic fields to regenerate peripheral nerves has recently been completed at Cornell University College of Medicine's Department of Obstetrics and Gynecology, Division of Reproductive Endocrinology. Under the direction of Dr. Brij Saxena, researchers demonstrated the successful growth and repair of cultured mice nerve cells using the Jacobson Resonator, invented by Dr. Jerry Jacobson of Jacobson Resonance Enterprises, in Boca Raton, Florida. In comparison to untreated controls, the treated nerves showed normal myelin sheaths and subcellular structures.[8]

Because most neurological disorders—Parkinson's disease, cerebral palsy, amyotrophic lateral sclerosis (Lou Gehrig's disease), multiple sclerosis, and so forth—are characterized by nerve damage, these findings are very exciting. The decline of multiple sclerosis patients, for example, is associated with the destruction of the protective myelin sheath that surrounds the nerves.

Saxena and colleagues are continuing their research in peripheral nerve regeneration with live mice. They have also performed a preliminary investigation of the effect of picotesla fields on the central nervous system (CNS). Using freshly autopsied human brain cells, the researchers were able to keep the treated cells alive longer than untreated samples.[9]

Other exciting neurological work is in progress using the Magnetic Molecular Energizing (MME) device, invented by Dr. Dean Bonlie of the Advanced Magnetic Research Institute in Calgary, Canada. In multiple clinical FDA trials in both Canada and the United States, researchers have reported dramatic improvement in patients suffering from a variety of neurological disorders—including Parkinson's disease, stroke, cranial nerve dysfunction, cerebral palsy, and multiple sclerosis—with the application of very strong direct-current electromagnetic fields targeting the brain. There has even been preliminary success with regaining some function in patients with spinal cord injuries.[10] When Superman (a.k.a. Christopher Reeve) insists that he'll walk again—this may be how he and many other quadriplegics will do it!

IN THE NEXT DECADE OR TWO

Within the next decade, we will have many more questions answered about the most efficacious use of static magnets for self-treatment. We will also have access to electromagnetic healing devices. The Jacobson Resonator is nearing final FDA approval for the treatment of osteoarthritis of the knee. As mentioned in the preceding section, the MME is currently undergoing

FDA clinical trials. Once a device is approved for one condition, it can then be used for many others. Approximately 60 percent of all pharmaceuticals in this country are currently used for "off-label" purposes.[11] So once these devices are FDA-approved, a whole new world of healing possibilities will open up.

When I listen to the accounts of remarkable case histories presented by dedicated researchers and clinicians, it sounds like science fiction. But soon it will be "science fact." In the next decade or two, energy medicine—including magnetic healing—will become part and parcel of this country's medical cornucopia. What is incurable today may very well be healed by magnet therapy tomorrow.

APPENDIX I

RESOURCES

Magnetic Product Distributors

ALBERT ROY DAVIS
RESEARCH LABS
P.O. Box 655
Green Cove Springs, FL
32043
(904) 264-8564

AMERICAN HEALTH SERVICE
MAGNETICS
14092 Lambs Lane
Libertyville, IL 60048
(800) 635-7070
(847) 573-8750

AMERIFLEX, INC.
232 N.E. Lincoln St., Suite G
Hillsboro, OR 97124
(800) 487-5463
(503) 640-0810

BEFIT ENTERPRISES, LTD.
The Cutting Edge Catalog
P.O. Box 5034
Southampton, NY 11969
(800) 497-9516
(516) 287-3813
www.cutcat.com

BIOMAGNETIC RESOURCES
539 Accord Sta.
Accord, MA 02018
(800) 890-3618
(781) 340-1072
www.biomagnetic.com

BODY MAGNETICS PLUS
871 Thrall Ave.
Suffield, CT 06078
(888) 668-5137
(860) 668-5137

BUY-A-MAG COMPANY
336 N. Coast Highway 101
Encintas, CA 92024
(800) 686-5232
(760) 943-0960

COMTRAD INDUSTRIES
2820 Waterford Lake Dr.,
Suite 102
Midlothian, VA 28113
(800) 704-1211
(804) 744-7155
www.comtrad.com

DENDEE INTERNATIONAL
P.O. Box 106
Clearlake, IA 50428
(515) 357-7893

ENVIRO-TECH PRODUCTS
(Philpott)
17171 S.E. 29th St.
Choctaw, OK 73020
(800) 445-1962

HOMEDICS, INC.
(In some chain drug and
department stores)
3000 Pontiac Trail
Commerce Township, MI
48390
(800) 333-8282
(248) 863-3000
www.homedics.com

HSW SYSTEMS
1027 S. Rainbow Blvd.
Las Vegas, NV 89128
(800) 793-3757
www.solutions.com

THE HUMAN TOUCH
2280 Grass Valley Hwy.,
Suite 130
Auburn, CA 95603
(888) 262-6252

JAPAN LIFE
(Multilevel Marketing
Company)
1025 Bedmar St.
Carson, CA 90746
(800) 877-5542
(310) 608-1311

KHT SYSTEMS
Korean Hand Therapy
P.O. Box 5309
Hemet, CA 92544
(877) 244-4352
(909) 766-1426
www.khtsystems.com

LGS TRUST
Lyon Magnetic Health
Products
P.O. Box 248
Holmen, WI 54636
(800) 778-5731
(608) 526-2178
www.lgstrust.com

MAGNABLOC
7575 Fulton St. E.
Building 33A2L
Ada, MI 49355
(877) 624-6225
www.magnabloc.com

MAGNESPORT
806 W. Diamond Ave.,
Suite 200
Gaithersburg, MD 20878
(800) 525-0644
(301) 738-7756
www.magnesport.com

MAGNETHERAPY, INC.
(Markov)
Tectonic Magnets
950 Congress Ave.
Rivera Beach, FL 33404-
6400
(800) 625-9736
(516) 882-0092
www.das-mall.com/tectonic

MAGNETICO., INC. (Bonlie)
No. 107, 5421 11th St. NE
Calgary, Alberta T2E 6M4
Canada
(800) 265-1119
(403) 730-0883
www.magneticosleep.com

MAGNETIC THERAPEUTIC
TECHNOLOGY, INC.
1915 Peters Rd., Suite 106
Irving, TX 75061
(800) 371-1113
(972) 721-9227
www.mplusmagnet.com

MAGNETIC WELLNESS
CENTER
P.O. Box 478
New York, NY 10002
(877) 602-1012
(646) 602-1012
www.magnetwell.com

MAGNETIC WELLNESS
PRODUCTS, INC.
3500 Parkdale Ave., Bldg. A
Baltimore, MD 21211
(800) 296-4660
www.magwellness.com

MID-AMERICAN MARKETING
P.O. Box 295
Eaton, OH 45320
(800) 922-1744
(937) 456-9393

NIKKEN, INC. (Multilevel
Marketing Company)
North American
Headquarters
15363 Barranca Pkwy.
Irvine, CA 92618
(888) 2-NIKKEN
www.nikken.com

NORSO BIOMAGNETICS, INC.
8724B Glenwood Ave.
Raleigh, NC 27612
(800) 480-8601
(919) 783-5911
www.promagnet.com

NUENERGY MAGNETICS
809 Lakeshore Blvd., R.R. I
Sauble Beach, Ontario N0H
2G0
Canada
(800) 544-0437

PAIN STOPS HERE, INC.
100 Fox Hill Dr.
Baiting Hollow, NY 11933
(888) 933-6400
www.magnetic-force.com

PJAN INTERNATIONAL, INC.
P.O. Box 1692
Stow, OH 44224
(800) 438-7736
www.magnetsolutions.com

POST INTERNATIONAL
P.O. Box 788
Roy, WA 98580
(253) 843-1321

PSYCHOPHYSICSLABS (Payne)
4264 Topsail Ct.
Soquel, CA 95037
(408) 462-1588

R.D.G. TECHNOLOGIES, INC.
913 9th Terr.
Palm Beach Gardens, FL
33418
(407) 625-0462

RUCK ENTERPRISES, INC.
650 W. Grand Ave., Unit 110
Elmhurst, IL 60126
(800) 366-7825

SBJ ENTERPRISES
6012 S. Linden Road, No. 18
Swartz Creek, MI 48472
(810) 655-2000
www.sbjenterprisesinc.com

SERENITY 2000
99 Telson Rd.
Markham, Ontario L3R 1E4
Canada
(800) 461-6398
(905) 470-2270
www.serenity.com

SPI, INC.
400 St. Paul St., Suite 1400
Dallas, TX 75201
(800) 322-0688
(214) 740-9797
www.spiinc-tx.com

TENGAM (Nellessen)
4957 Bittrich-Antler Rd.
Deer Park, WA 99006
(509) 276-2054

WHEATLEY HEALTH
PRODUCTS
585 Dean St.
Brooklyn, NY 11238
(800) 951-7246

WONDER COMFORTS
INTERNATIONAL
BIOflex
2633 Lincoln Blvd., Suite 435
Santa Monica, CA 90405
(888) 334-2000
(310) 306-3489
www.magneticproducts.com

Magnet Therapy

Organizations/Training Programs

AMERICAN UNIVERSITY OF COMPLEMENTARY MEDICINE
11543 Olympic Blvd.
Los Angeles, CA 90064
(310) 914-4116
www.aucm.org

   AUCM offers California state-approved graduate degrees and certificate programs in complementary and alternative medicine, with course work including energy medicine techniques. A 60-hour segment in biomagnetic therapy may be audited, taken separately and/or is available for continuing education credits.

BIO-ELECTRIC-MAGNETICS INSTITUTE (BEMI)
2940 W. Moana Ln.
Reno, NV 89509-7801
(775) 827-9099

BEMI is an IRS-registered 501(c)(3) nonprofit research and educational organization, founded in 1986 by Dr. John Zimmerman. Its informational packet, available for a $10 donation, contains lists of distributors and practitioners, a comparison of magnetic bed products, a glossary of biomagnetic terms, and additional background material on magnet therapy.

BIOELECTROMAGNETICS SOCIETY
P.O. Box 3651
Arlington, VA 22203
(703) 524-2367
www.bioelectromagnetics.org

The Bioelectromagnetics Society sponsors conferences and distributes a newsletter devoted to current issues in bioelectromagnetics.

HEALTHWORLD ONLINE
4215 Glencoe Ave.
Marina del Rey, CA 90292
(310) 821-0222
www.healthy.net/biomagnetics

HealthWorld Online is a comprehensive global health network on the Internet. Its Center for Biomagnetic and Electromagnetic Field Resources provides information resources (news, reviews, research abstracts, articles, educational opportunities, and a calendar of presentations), services (speakers' network and cybrarian service), and product and books.

KHT Systems
P.O. Box 5309
Hemet, CA 92544
(877) 244-4352
(909) 766-1426
www.khtsystems.com

KHT Systems provides training tapes, books, supplies (including point magnets), and workshops on Korean Hand Therapy (KHT).

North American Academy of Magnetic Therapy
P.O. Box 447
Agoura Hills, CA 91376-0447
(818) 991-5277
www.naamt.org

NAAMT presents an annual conference (January) on recent biomagnetic scientific research, clinical studies, and therapeutic applications—continuing education credits available. Call for conference tapes and abstracts. It also offers a training program for health-care practitioners and is in the process of establishing product standards.

APPENDIX 2

SELECTED MAGNET THERAPY
ACUPUNCTURE POINTS

Some Helpful Points

Ankle pain: GB 40, K 6
Elbow pain: LI 11
Headache: B 2, GB 20, GV 24.5, LI 4
Knee pain: B 54, ST 36, LV 8
Lower back pain: B 22–B 25
Menstrual pain: C 4, C 6, SP 12, SP 13
Neck pain: B 2, B 10, GB 20
Shoulder pain: GB 20, GB 21, TW 15
Wrist pain: P 6, P 7, TW 4, TW 5

Point Locations

All points are bilateral, except C 4, C 6, and GV 24.5.
Do not use GB 21 or LI 4 if you are pregnant.

Bladder Meridian (B)

B 2: Where the bridge of the nose meets the inner ridge of the eyebrows at the indentation of each inner eye socket.

B 10: On the ropy muscles one-half inch away from the spine and about one-half inch below the base of the skull.

B 22–B 25: Two finger-widths from the spine, starting at the waist and extending downward 2 to 4 inches.

B 54: In the center of the crease of the knee joint.

Conception Vessel Meridian (C)

C 4: Four finger-widths below the navel.

C 6: Two finger-widths below the navel.

Gallbladder Meridian (GB)

GB 20: In the hollow, approximately 2 to 3 inches wide, between the two large vertical neck muscles below the base of the skull.

GB 21: On the highest point of the shoulder muscle, 1 to 2 inches from either side of the base of the neck. *Do not use if pregnant.*

GB 40: Directly in front of the outer anklebone, in the large hollow.

Governing Vessel Meridian (GV)

GV 24.5: Between the eyebrows where the bridge of the nose meets the forehead.

Kidney Meridian (K)

K 6: One thumb-width directly below the inner anklebone.

Large Intestine (LI)

LI 4: At the highest spot on the muscle in the webbing between the thumb and index finger. *Do not use if pregnant.*

LI 11: At the upper edge of the outer elbow crease.

Liver Meridian (LV)

LV 8: Where the crease ends on the inner side of the knee when it is bent.

Pericardium (P)

P 6: Two and one-half finger-widths above the wrist crease in the middle of the inner forearm.

P 7: In the middle of the inner wrist crease.

Spleen (SP)

SP 12: In the middle of the crease where the leg joins the body trunk.

SP 13: One finger-width above SP 12 and a little toward the hip.

Stomach (ST)

ST 36: One finger-width outside of the shinbone, four finger-widths below the kneecap.

Triple Warmer (TW)

TW 4: In the hollow of the center of the outer wrist crease.

TW 5: Two and one-half finger-widths above the outer wrist crease.

TW 15: One-half inch below the top of the shoulder, midway between the base of the neck and the outer edge of the shoulder.

GV 24.5

B 2 —— —— B 2

LI 11 —— —— LI 11

C 6
C 4

SP 13 SP 13
SP 12 SP 12

LI 4 —— —— LI 4

LV 8 —— —— LV 8
ST 36 —— —— ST 36

K 6 —— —— GB 40

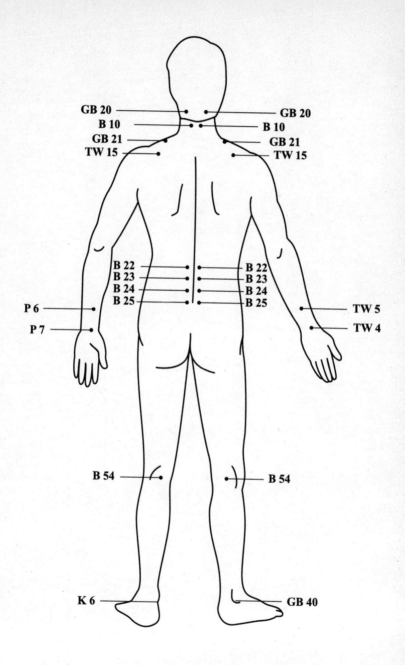

APPENDIX 3

KOREAN HAND THERAPY OVERVIEW

Treating Front of Body

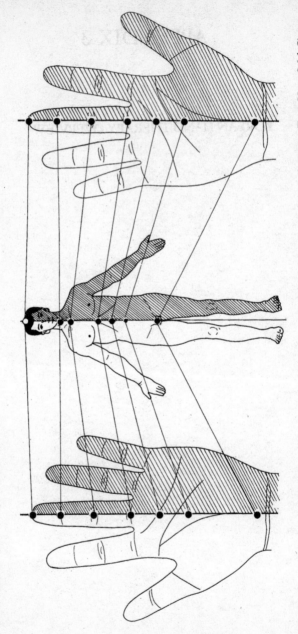

Source: Reprinted with permission from T. W. Yoo, *Koryo Hands Acupuncture,* vol. I (Seoul, Korea: Eum Yang Mek Jin Publishing Co., 1988), 71–72.

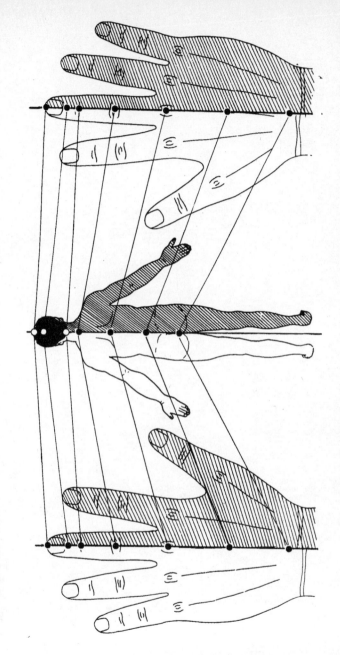

Treating Back of Body

NOTES

CHAPTER 1. AN ANCIENT TOOL FOR MODERN TIMES

1. Abstracts from the Second World Congress for Electricity and Magnetism in Biology and Medicine (1997). Obtained from: http://info-ventures.com/emf/meetings/bems.

2. R. Lawrence, P. J. Rosch, and J. Plowden, *Magnet Therapy: The Pain Cure Alternative* (Rocklin, Calif.: Prima Health, 1998), 70, 101–102.

3. R. O. Becker and G. Selden, *The Body Electric: Electromagnetism and the Foundation of Life* (New York: Morrow, 1985), 244–45.

4. H. Hannemann, *Magnet Therapy: Balancing Your Body's Energy Flow for Self-Healing* (New York: Sterling, 1990), 17.

5. A. Cox, "Magnetic Field Reversals," *Scientific American,* February 1967, 44–54; D. Gubbins and J. Bloxhan, "The Secular Variation of the Earth's Magnetic Field," *Nature,* 317 (October 31, 1985).

6. K. Nakagawa, "Magnetic Field Deficiency Syndrome and Magnetic Treatment," *Japanese Medical Journal* 2745, (December 4, 1976).

7. Hannemann, *Magnet Therapy,* 59.

CHAPTER 2. THE HISTORY OF MAGNET THERAPY

1. A. M. Schoen, *Veterinary Acupuncture: Ancient Art to Modern Medicine* (Goleta, Calif.: American Veterinarian Publications, 1994).

2. R. O. Becker, *Cross Currents: The Promise of Electromedicine, the Perils of Electropollution* (Los Angeles: Tarcher, 1990), 14.

3. G. Washins, *Discovery of Magnetic Health* (Rockville, Md.: Nova Publishing), 200.

4. Becker, *Cross Currents*, 17.

5. R. Miller, "Methods of Detecting and Measuring Healing Energies," in *Future Science*, edited by J. W. White and S. Krippner, 431–44 (Garden City, N.Y.: Doubleday, 1977).

6 J. Carper, *Miracle Cures* (New York: HarperCollins, 1998), 14.

7. Ibid., 92.

8. Ibid., 135.

CHAPTER 3. THE NATURE OF MAGNETS

1. R. O. Becker, *Cross Currents: The Promise of Electromedicine, The Perils of Electropollution* (Los Angeles: Tarcher, 1990), 173–184.

2. R. O. Becker and G. Selden, *The Body Electric: Electromagnetism and the Foundation of Life* (New York: Morrow, 1985), 252–55.

3. Ibid., 254.

4. R. Sandyk, P. A. Anninos, and N. Tsagas, "Magnetic Fields and Seasonality of Affective Illness: Implications for Therapy," *International Journal of Neuroscience* 58, nos. 3–4 (1991): 261–67.

5. J. Zimmerman, "Laying-On-of-Hands Healing and Therapeutic Touch: A Testable Theory," *Newsletter of the Bio-Electro-Magnetics Institute* 2, no. 1 (spring 1990), 7–18.

6. M. Feychting and A. Ahlbom, "Childhood Leukemia and Residential Exposure to Weak Extremely Low Frequency Magnetic Fields," *Environmental Health Perspectives* 103, suppl. 2 (1995): 59–62.

7.   R. P. Liburdy et al., "ELF Magnetic Fields, Breast Cancer, and Melatonin: 60 Hz Fields Block Melatonin's Oncostatic Action on ER+ Breast Cancer Cell Proliferation," *Journal of Pineal Research* 14, no. 2 (1993): 89–97.

8.   National Institutes of Health/National Cancer Institute, "62991-02 EMF and Breast Cancer" (1997). Obtained from www.epa.gov/edrlupvx/inventory/NCE018.html.

9.   Abstracts from the Second World Congress for Electricity and Magnetism in Biology and Medicine (1997). Obtained from http://info-ventures.com/emf/meetings/bems.

10.   ReutersHealth/MedNews, "Mobile Telephone Use May Be Associated with Headaches, Fatigue" (May 19, 1998); obtained from: www.reutershealth.mednews. B. Hocking, "Preliminary Report: Symptoms Associated with Mobile Phone Use," *Occupational Medicine* 48, no. 6 (1998): 357–60.

11.   S. Braune et al., "Resting Blood Pressure Increases during Exposure to a Radio-Frequency Electromagnetic Field," *Lancet* 351 (1998): 1857–58.

12.   H. Resier, W. Dimpfel, and F. Schober, "The Influence of Electromagnetic Fields on Human Brain Activity," *European Journal of Medical Research* 1, no. 1 (1995): 27–32.

13.   K. Mann and J. Roschke, "Effects of Pulsed High-Frequency Electromagnetic Fields on Human Sleep," *Neuropsychobiology* 33, no. 1 (1996): 41–47.

14.   A. L. Galeev, "Effects of the Microwave Radiation from the

Cellular Phones on Humans and Animals," *Ross Fiziol Zh Im I M Sechenova* 84, no. 11 (1998): 1293–1302.

15. S. Kahn, *The Nurse's Meditative Journal* (Albany, N.Y.: Delmar, 1996), 23.

16. R. C. Beck, "Mood Modification with ELF Magnetic Fields: A Preliminary Exploration," *Archaeus* 4 (1986): 48.

CHAPTER 4. HOW MAGNETS HEAL

1. "Acupuncture NIH Consensus Statement Online," November 3–5, 1997. Obtained from http://opd.od.nih.gov/consensus/cons/107/107_statement.htm.

2. S. Liss, "Effects of Magnets and Other Electrical Stimulation Devices on Human Serum Chemistry" (paper presented at the fifth annual meeting of the North American Academy of Magnetic Therapy, Los Angeles, January 22–24, 1999), audiotape.

3. T. J. Kaptchuk, *The Web That Has No Weaver* (New York: Condon & Weed, 1983), 80.

4. E. R. Sanseverino, A. Vannini, and P. Castellaci, "Therapeutic Effects of Pulsed Magnetic Fields on Joint Disease," *Panminerva Med* 34, no. 4 (1992): 187–96.

5. R. Lawrence, P. J. Rosch, and J. Plowden, *Magnet Therapy: The Pain Cure Alternative* (Rocklin, Calif.: Prima Health, 1998), 134.

6. W. Philpott and S. L. Taplin, *Biomagnetic Handbook: Today's Introduction to the Energy Medicine of Tomorrow* (Choctaw, Okla.: Enviro-Tech Products, 1990), 24.

7. A. R. Davis and W. Rawls, *The Magnetic Effect* (Kansas City, Mo.: Acres USA, 1975); A. R. Davis and W. Rawls, *The Magnetic Blueprint of Life* (Kansas City, Mo.: Acres USA, 1979).

8. R. Karabakhtsian et al., "Calcium Is Necessary in the Cell Response to Electromagnetic Fields," *FEBS Letter* 349, no. 1 (1994): 1–6.

9. A. Cox, "Magnetic Field Reversals," *Scientific American*, February 1967, 44–54; D. Gubbins and J. Bloxhan, "The Secular Variation of the Earth's Magnetic Field," *Nature* 317 (October 31, 1985).

10. K. Nakagawa, "Magnetic Field Deficiency Syndrome and Magnetic Treatment," *Japanese Medical Journal* 2745 (December 4, 1976).

11. J. Smith, "The Influence on Enzyme Growth by the 'Laying on of Hands,'" in *The Dimensions of Healing: A Symposium* (Los Altos, Calif.: Academy of Parapsychology and Medicine, 1972).

12. L-S. Gao, "The Effect of Magnetized Water on Digestive Enzymes," Department of Biology, Guangdong College of Education, Guangzhou, China.

13. Liss, "Effects of Magnets."

14. R. Miller, "Methods of Detecting and Measuring Healing Energies," in *Future Science*, edited by J. W. White and S. Krippner, 431–44 (Garden City, N.Y.: Doubleday, 1977).

15. Jacobson Resonance Enterprises, "Jacobson Resonance Enterprises, Inc., Announces Texas A&M Study Demonstrates Magnetized Water May Enhance Growth of Squash," *PR Newswire*, January 19, 1999.

16. Smith, "Influence on Enzyme Growth"; Gao, "Effect of Magnetized Water."

17. J. Wu, "Further Observations on the Therapeutic Effect of Magnets and Magnetized Water against Ascariasis in Children—Analysis of 114 Cases," *Journal of Traditional Chinese Medicine* 2 (1989): 111–12.

CHAPTER 5. LOOKING AT THE EVIDENCE

1. D. M. Eisenberg et al., "Trends in Alternative Medicine Use in the United States, 1990–1997: Results of a Follow-up National Survey," *Journal of the American Medical Association* 280 (1998): 1569–75.

2. J. Carper, *Miracle Cures* (New York: HarperCollins, 1998), 26.

3. S. Liss, "Effects of Magnets and Other Electrical Stimulation Devices on Human Serum Chemistry" (paper presented at the fifth annual meeting of the North American Academy of Magnetic Therapy, Los Angeles, January 22–24, 1999), audiotape.

4. H. Hannemann, *Magnet Therapy: Balancing Your Body's Energy Flow for Self-Healing* (New York: Sterling Publishing, 1990), 16.

5. Ibid.

6. T. Laser, "Double-Blind Study of the Therapeutic Effectiveness of Permanently Magnetized Foils on Secondary Myotendo-fasciopathies at Different Selected Locations." Obtained from www.magneticproducts.com/ms5.htm.

7. J. Zimmerman, "Double-Blind Placebo-Controlled Study of Permanent Magnets for the Treatment of Low Back Pain" (paper pre-

sented at the fifth annual meeting of the North American Academy of Magnetic Therapy, Los Angeles, January 22–24, 1999), audiotape.

8. D. Foley-Nolan et al., "Pulsed High Frequency (27 MHz) Electromagnetic Therapy for Persistent Neck Pain," *Orthopedics* 13, no. 4 (1990): 445–51.

9. E. A. Ghoname, W. Craig, W. F. White, et al., "Percutaneous Electrical Nerve Stimulation for Low Back Pain: A Randomized Crossover Study," *Journal of the American Medical Association* 281, no. 9 (1999): 818–23.

10. C. A. Bassett, "Fundamental and Practical Aspects of Therapeutic Uses of Pulsed Electromagnetic Fields (PEMFs)," *Critical Reviews in Biomedical Engineering* 17, no. 5 (1989): 451–529.

11. J. Jerabek and W. Pawluk, *Magnetic Therapy in Eastern Europe: A Review of 30 Years of Research* (William Pawluk, wpawluk@ compuserve.com, 1998), 92–93.

12. Ibid., 81–82.

13. Ibid., 56.

14. M. J. McLean et al., "Treatment of Wrist Pain in the Work Place with a Static Magnetic Device—Interim Report of a Clinical Trial" (paper presented at the Second World Congress for Electricity and Magnetism in Biology and Medicine, Bologna, Italy, June 8–13, 1997).

15. Jerabek and Pawluk, *Magnetic Therapy in Eastern Europe*, 65.

16. R. Lawrence, P. J. Rosch, and J. Plowden, *Magnet Therapy: The Pain Cure Alternative* (Rocklin, Calif.: Prima Health, 1998), 132.

17. K. E. Johnson et al., "The Effectiveness of a Magnetized Water Oral Irrigator (Hydro Floss) on Plaque, Calculus and Gingival Health," *Journal of Clinical Periodontology* 25, no. 4 (1998): 316–21.

18. Jerabek and Pawluk, *Magnetic Therapy in Eastern Europe*, 73.

19. V. E. Kriokshina et al., "Use of Micromagnets in Stomatology," *Magnitologiia* 1 (1991): 17–20.

20. Jerabek and Pawluk, *Magnetic Therapy in Eastern Europe*, 71–73.

21. L. C. Rhodes, "The Adjunctive Utilization of Diapulse Therapy (Pulsed High Peak Power Electromagnetic Energy) in Accelerating Tissue Healing in Oral Surgery," *Quarterly of the National Dental Association* 40, no. 1 (1981): 4–11.

22. A. Pascual-Leone, et al., "Rapid-Rate Transcranial Magnetic Stimulation of Left Dorsolateral Prefrontal Cortex in Drug-Resistant Depression," *Lancet* 348, no. 9022 (1996): 233–37.

23. A. Conca et al., "Transcranial Magnetic Stimulation: A Novel Antidepressive Strategy?" *Neuropsychobiology* 34, no. 4 (1996): 204–7.

24. G. S. Figiel et al., "The Use of Rapid-Rate Transcranial Magnetic Stimulation (rTMS) in Refractory Depressed Patients," *Journal of Neuropsychiatry and Clinical Neuroscience* 10, no. 1 (1998): 20–25.

25. M. S. George et al., "Mood Improvement Following Daily Left Prefrontal Repetitive Transcranial Magnetic Stimulation in Patients with Depression: A Placebo-Controlled Crossover Trial," *American Journal of Psychiatry* 154 (1997): 1752–56.

26. M. S. George, S. H. Lisanby, and H. A. Sackeim, "Transcranial Magnetic Stimulation: Applications in Neuropsychiatry," *Archives of General Psychiatry* 56, no. 4 (1999): 300–311.

27. E. Klein et al., "Therapeutic Efficacy of Right Prefrontal Slow Repetitive Transcranial Magnetic Stimulation in Major Depression: A Double-Blind Controlled Study," *Archives of General Psychiatry* 56, no. 4 (1999): 315–20; V. Geller et al., "Slow Magnetic Stimulation of Prefrontal Cortex in Depression and Schizophrenia," *Progress in Neuropsychopharmacology and Biological Psychiatry* 21, no. 1 (1997): 105–10.

28. D. L. Menkes et al., "Right Frontal Lobe Slow Frequency Repetitive Transcranial Magnetic Stimulation (SF r-TMS) Is an Effective Treatment for Depression: A Case-Control Pilot Study of Safety and Efficacy," *Journal of Neurological and Neurosurgical Psychiatry* 67, no. 1 (1999): 113–15.

29. W. Philpott and S. L. Taplin, *Biomagnetic Handbook: Today's Introduction to the Energy Medicine of Tomorrow* (Choctaw, Okla.: Enviro-Tech Products, 1990), 46, 50, 83.

30. F. Tergau et al., "Low-Frequency Repetitive Transcranial Magnetic Stimulation Improves Intractable Epilepsy," *Lancet* 353, no. 9171 (1999): 2209.

31. P. A. Anninos et al., "Magnetic Stimulation in the Treatment of Partial Seizures," *International Journal of Neuroscience* 60, nos. 3–4 (1991): 141–71.

32. R. Sandyk and P. A. Anninos, "Magnetic Fields Alter the Circadian Periodicity of Seizures," *International Journal of Neuroscience* 63, nos. 3–4 (1992): 265–74.

33. Telephone conversation with Dr. Jerry Jacobson, Jacobson Resonance Enterprises, Boca Raton, Fla., June 17, 1999.

34. G. D. Antimonii and R. A. Salamov, "Action of a Modulated

Electromagnetic Field on Experimentally Induced Epileptiform Brain Activity in Rats," *Biull Eksp Biol Med*, 89, no. 2 (1980): 145–48.

35. M. J. McLean et al., "Therapeutic Efficacy of a Static Magnetic Device in Three Animal Seizure Models: Summary of Experience" (paper presented at the Second World Congress for Electricity and Magnetism in Biology and Medicine, Bologna, Italy, June 8–13, 1997).

36. Philpott and Taplin, *Biomagnetic Handbook*, 55.

37. Telephone conversation with Dr. Ellen Kamhi, Huntington, NY, June 14, 1999.

38. L. K. S. Kim, "The Effect of Magnetic Application for Primary Dysmenorrhea," *Kanhohak Tamgu* 3, no. 1 (1994): 148–73.

39. Jerabek and Pawluk, *Magnetic Therapy in Eastern Europe*, 67.

40. Telephone conversation with Dr. Kamhi, June 14, 1999.

41. Jerabek and Pawluk, *Magnetic Therapy in Eastern Europe*, 69–70.

42. M. Damirov et al., "Magnetic-Infrared-Laser-Therapeutic Apparatus (MILTA) in Treatment of Patients with Endometriosis," *Vrach* 12 (1994): 17–19.

43. G. Varcaddio-Garofalo et al., "Analgesic Properties of Electromagnetic Field Therapy in Patients with Chronic Pelvic Pain," *Clinical Experience in Obstetrics and Gynecology* 22, no. 4 (1995): 350–54.

44. Jerabek and Pawluk, *Magnetic Therapy in Eastern Europe*, 66.

45. Ibid., 69.

46. N. T. Galloway et al., "Extracorporeal Magnetic Innervation Therapy for Stress Urinary Incontinence," *Urology* 53, no. 6 (1999): 1108–11.

47. Lawrence, Rosch, and Plowden, *Magnet Therapy*, 175–76.

48. A. Gill Taylor, "A Center to Test the Efficacy of Static Magnetic Fields and Other Selected Complementary and Alternative Therapies" (paper presented at the fifth annual meeting of the North American Academy of Magnetic Therapy, Los Angeles, January 22–24, 1999), audiotape.

49. Telephone conversation with Dr. Kamhi, June 14, 1999.

50. M. I. Weintraub, "Chronic Submaximal Magnetic Stimulation in Peripheral Neuropathy: Is There a Beneficial Therapeutic Relationship?" *American Journal of Pain Management* 8 (1998): 12–16.

51. M. I. Weintraub, "Magnetic Bio-stimulation in Painful Diabetic Peripheral Neuropathy: A Novel Intervention—A Randomized, Double-Placebo Crossover Study," *American Journal of Pain Management* 9, no. 1 (1999): 8–17.

52. L. Seaman, "A Double-Blind Study Demonstrating Therapeutic Benefit in Heel Pain Symptomatology." Obtained from www.magnetic products.com/ms3.htm.

53. R. A. Sherman, L. Robson, and L. A. Marden, "Initial Exploration of Pulsing Electromagnetic Fields for Treatment of Migraine," *Headache* 38, no. 3 (1998): 208–13.

54. R. Sandyk, "The Influence of the Pineal Gland on Migraine and Cluster Headaches and Effects of Treatment with Picotesla Magnetic Fields," *International Journal of Neuroscience* 67, nos. 1–4 (1992): 145–71.

55. A. Prusinksi et al., "Pulsating Electromagnetic Field in the Therapy of Headache" (paper presented at the Hungarian

Symposium on Magnetotherapy, Szekesfehervar, Hungary, May 16–17, 1987), 163–66.

56. L. Lazar and A. Farago, "Experiences of Patients Suffering from Migraine-Type Headache Treated with Magnetotherapy" (paper presented at the Hungarian Symposium on Magnetotherapy, Szekesfehervar, Hungary, May 16–17, 1987), 137–40.

57. J. Giczi and A. Guseo, "Treatment of Headache with Pulsating Electromagnetic Field: A Preliminary Report" (paper presented at the Hungarian Symposium on Magnetotherapy, Szekesfehervar, Hungary, May 16–17, 1987), 74–76.

58. Jerabek and Pawluk, *Magnetic Therapy in Eastern Europe*, 35.

59. B. M. Popov and T. A. Al'shanskaya, "Use of Traditional and Nontraditional Methods in the Treatment of Headaches," in *Millimeter Waves in Medicine and Biology*, digest of papers of the eleventh Russian Symposium with International Participation, Zvenigorod, Moscow Region, Russia, April 21–24, 1997, 68–71.

60. Telephone conversation with Dr. Kamhi, June 14, 1999.

61. Philpott and Taplin, *Biomagnetic Handbook*, 62.

62. Jerabek and Pawluk, *Magnetic Therapy in Eastern Europe*, 26.

63. S. G. Ivanov, "The Comparative Efficacy of Nondrug and Drug Methods of Treating Hypertension," *Ter Arkh* 65, no. 1 (1993): 44–49.

64. Telephone conversation with Dr. Xiu Ling Ma, September 12, 1999.

65. Telephone conversation with Tom Nellessen, July 13, 1999.

66. S. G. Ivanov et al., "Use of Magnetic Fields in the Treatment of Hypertensive Disease," *Vopr Kurotol Fizioter Lech Fiz Kult* 3 (1993): 67–69.

67. Jacobson Resonance Enterprises, "Preliminary Data from University of Oklahoma Studies Provide Strong Evidence That the Jacobson Resonator Can Noninvasively Regulate Heart Rate in Dogs," *Newswire,* May 20, 1999.

68. G. Guilleminault and B. Pasche, "Clinical Effects of Low Energy Emission Therapy for Treatment of Insomnia" (paper presented at the fifteenth annual meeting of the Bioelectromagnetics Society, Los Angeles, June 13–17, 1993), 84; M. Erman et al., "Low-Energy Emission Therapy (LEET) Treatment for Insomnia" (paper presented at the thirteenth annual meeting of the Bioelectromagnetics Society, Salt Lake City, June 23–27, 1991), 69.

69. Telephone conversation with Dr. Ma, September 12, 1999.

70. R. Sandyk, "Rapid Normalization of Visual Evoked Potentials: Picotesla Range Magnetic Fields in Chronic Progressive Multiple Sclerosis," *International Journal of Neuroscience* 77, nos. 3–4 (1994): 243–59; R. Sandyk, "Progressive Cognitive Improvement in Multiple Sclerosis from Treatment with Electromagnetic Fields," *International Journal of Neuroscience* 89, nos. 1–2 (1997): 39–51; R. Sandyk, "Treatment with Electromagnetic Field Alters the Clinical Course of Chronic Progressive Multiple Sclerosis—A Case Report," *International Journal of Neuroscience* 88, nos. 1–2 (1996): 75–82; R. Sandyk, "Treatment with Weak Electromagnetic Fields Improves Fatigue Associated with Multiple Sclerosis," *International Journal of Neuroscience,* 84, nos. 1–4 (1996): 177–86.

71. A. Guseo, "Double-Blind Treatments with Pulsating Electromagnetic Field in Multiple Sclerosis" (paper presented at the

Hungarian Symposium on Magnetotherapy, Szekesfehervar, Hungary, May 16–17, 1987), 85–89.

72. A. Sieron et al., "The Variable Magnetic Fields in the Complex Treatment of Neurological Diseases" (paper presented at the European Bioelectromagnetics Association, Third Internal Congress, Nancy, France, February 29–March 3, 1996).

73. L. Pearce, "Clinical Experience with a High Strength Static Magnetic Field in Neurological Practice" (paper presented at the fifth annual meeting of the North American Academy of Magnetic Therapy, Los Angeles, January 22–24, 1999), audiotape.

74. Telephone conversation with Dr. David Stokesbary, September 9, 1999.

75. D. H. Trock et al., "A Double-Blind Trial of the Clinical Effects of Pulsed Electromagnetic Fields in Osteoarthritis," *Journal of Rheumatology* 20, no. 3 (1993): 456–60.

76. D. H. Trock, A. J. Bollet, and R. Markoll, "The Effect of Pulsed Electromagnetic Fields in the Treatment of Osteoarthritis of the Knee and Cervical Spine: Report of Randomized, Double-Blind, Placebo-Controlled Trials," *Journal of Rheumatology* 10 (1994): 1903–11.

77. T. M. Zizic et al., "The Treatment of Osteoarthritis of the Knee with Pulsed Electrical Stimulation," *Journal of Rheumatology* 22, no. 9 (1995): 1757–61.

78. Telephone conversation with Dr. Jacobson, June 17, 1999.

79. C. Hershler, "Pulsed Signal Therapy of Osteoarthritis and Soft Tissue Injury" (paper presented at the fifth annual meeting of the

North American Academy of Magnetic Therapy, Los Angeles, January 22–24, 1999), audiotape.

80.   R. Lawrence, P. J. Rosch, and J. Plowden, *Magnet Therapy: The Pain Care Alternative* (Rocklin, Calif.: Prima Health, 1998), 95.

81.   Telephone conversation with Dr. Kamhi, June 14, 1999.

82.   R. Sandyk, "Magnetic Fields in the Therapy of Parkinsonism," *International Journal of Neuroscience* 66, nos. 3–4 (1992): 209–35; R. Sandyk, "A Drug Naïve Parkinsonian Patient Successfully Treated with Weak Electromagnetic Fields," *International Journal of Neuroscience* 79, nos. 1–2 (1994): 99–110; R. Sandyk and K. Derpapas, "The Effects of External Picotesla Range Magnetic Fields on the EEG in Parkinson's Disease," *International Journal of Neuroscience* 70, nos. 1–2 (1993): 85–96.

83.   M. S. George et al., "Transcranial Magnetic Stimulation: A Neuropsychiatric Tool for the 21st Century," *Journal of Neuropsychiatry and Clinical Neuroscience* 8, no. 4 (1996): 373–82.

84.   Pearce, "Clinical Experience with a High Strength Magnetic Field."

85.   C. Vallbona, C. F. Hazlewood, and F. Jurida, "Response of Pain to Static Magnetic Fields in Post-polio Patients: A Double-Blind Pilot Study," *Archives of Physical Medicine and Rehabilitation* 78, no. 11 (1997): 1200–1203.

86.   Jerabek and Pawluk, *Magnetic Therapy in Eastern Europe,* 44–45.

87.   Ibid., 139.

88.   Ibid., 47; H. Mohamed-Ali, "Influence of Electromagnetic

Fields on the Enzyme Activity of Rheumatoid Synovial Fluid Cells in Vitro," *European Journal of Clinical Chemistry and Clinical Biochemistry* 32, no. 4 (1994): 319–26.

89.   Jerabek and Pawluk, *Magnetic Therapy in Eastern Europe*, 52.

90.   G. Null, *Healing with Magnets* (New York: Carroll & Graf, 1998), 37.

91.   Ibid., 61.

92.   Telephone conversation with Jules Klapper, Cutting Edge Catalogue, Southampton, NY, July 14, 1999.

93.   H. Hannemann, *Magnet Therapy: Balancing Your Body's Energy Flow for Self-Healing* (New York: Sterling, 1990), 16.

94.   Telephone conversation with Dr. Stokesbary, September 9, 1999.

95.   J. Pujol et al., "The Effect of Repetitive Magnetic Stimulation on Localized Musculoskeletal Pain," *Neuroreport* 9, no. 8 (1998): 1745–48.

96.   A. A. Pila and L. Kloth, "Effect of Pulsed Radio Frequency Therapy on Edema in Ankle Sprains: A Multisite Double-Blind Clinical Study" (paper presented at the Second World Congress for Electricity and Magnetism in Biology and Medicine, Bologna, Italy, June 8–13, 1997), 300.

97.   A. Binder et al., "Pulsed Electromagnetic Field Therapy of Persistent Rotator Cuff Tendinitis: A Double-Blind Controlled Assessment," *Lancet* 1, no. 8379 (1984): 695–98.

98.   D. Foley-Nolan, "Low Energy High Frequency Pulsed Electromagnetic Therapy for Acute Whiplash Injuries: A Double-

Blind Randomized Controlled Study," *Scandanavian Journal of Rehabilitation Medicine* 24, no. I (1992): 51–59.

99. Jerabek and Pawluk, *Magnetic Therapy in Eastern Europe*, 63.

100. Ibid., 53.

101. Ibid., 65.

102. Ibid., 67.

103. D. Man et al., "Effect of Permanent Magnetic Field on Postoperative Pain and Wound Healing in Plastic Surgery" (paper presented at the Second World Congress for Electricity and Magnetism in Biology and Medicine, Bologna, Italy, June 8–13, 1997).

104. Jerabek and Pawluk, *Magnetic Therapy in Eastern Europe*, 68.

105. Jerabek and Pawluk, *Magnetic Therapy in Eastern Europe*, 64.

106. Ibid.

107. Ibid.

108. J. K. Szor and R. Topp, "Use of Magnet Therapy to Heal an Abdominal Wound: A Case Study," *Ostomy Wound Management* 44, no. 5 (1998): 24–29.

109. P. Kokoschinegg, "The Application of Static Alternating Magnetic Field in Medicine." Obtained from www.magneticproducts.com/ms6.htm.

CHAPTER 6. CHOOSING MAGNETS

I. F. Rinker, *The Invisible Force: Traditional Magnetic Therapy* (London, Ontario, Canada: Mason Service Publishing, 1997), 32–33.

2. World Health Organization, "Environmental Health Criteria, Magnetic Fields, 1987." Obtained from www.who.int.

3. J. Zimmerman, *Glossary of Terms and Conventions as Used in Magnetotherapy* (Reno, Nev.: Bio-Electro-Magnetics Institute, 1999), 2.

CHAPTER 7. TREATING WITH MAGNETS

1. J. Jerabek and W. Pawluk, *Magnetic Therapy in Eastern Europe: A Review of 30 Years of Research* (William Pawluk, wpawluk@compuserve.com, 1998): 137–38.

2. Telephone conversation with Dr. Xiu Ling Ma, September 12, 1999.

3. R. Lawrence, "Introduction—Questions and Answers" (paper presented at the fifth annual meeting of the North American Academy of Magnetic Therapy, Los Angeles, January 22–24, 1999), audiotape.

4. Telephone conversation with Dr. Ellen Kahmi, June 14, 1999.

5. H. Hannemann, *Magnet Therapy: Balancing Your Body's Energy Flow for Self-Healing* (New York: Sterling, 1990), 30–34.

6. Telephone conversation with Dr. Buryl Payne, July 16, 1999.

7. Telephone conversation with Tom Nellessen, July 13, 1999.

8. M. Markov, "Why Dosimetry of Magnetic Fields Is Important for Magnetic Therapy" (paper presented at the fifth annual meeting of the North American Academy of Magnetic Therapy, Los Angeles, January 22–24, 1999), audiotape.

9. P. E. Baldry, *Acupuncture, Trigger Points and Musculoskeletal Pain* (Edinburgh, Scotland: Churchill Livingstone, 1993), 96.

10.   T. J. Kaptchuk, *The Web That Has No Weaver* (New York: Congdon & Weed, 1983), 80.

11.   "Acupuncture: NIH Consensus Statement Online," November 3–5, 1997. Obtained from http://opd.od.nih.gov/consensus/cons/107/107_statement.htm.

12.   M. R. Gach, *Acupressure's Potent Points: A Guide to Self-Care for Common Ailments* (New York: Bantam Books, 1990).

13.   Jerabek and Pawluk, *Magnetic Therapy in Eastern Europe*, 136.

CHAPTER 8. AROUND THE CORNER

1.   A. Gill Taylor, "Controlled Clinical Trial of Two Different Magnetic Mattresses on Fibromyalgia" (paper presented at the sixth annual meeting of the North American Academy of Magnetic Therapy, Los Angeles, January 21–23, 2000).

2.   A. Colbert, "Magnetic Therapy Using Acupuncture Principles, Including Treatment of Depression" (paper presented at the sixth annual meeting of the North American Academy of Magnetic Therapy, Los Angeles, January 21–23, 2000).

3.   J. Zimmerman, "Follow-Up on Double-Blind, Placebo-Controlled Study of Permanent Magnets for the Treatment of Low Back Pain" (paper presented at the sixth annual meeting of the North American Academy of Magnetic Therapy, Los Angeles, January 21–23, 2000).

4.   R. Hottentot, "Use of Static Magnets in Orthopedics" (paper presented at the sixth annual meeting of the North American Academy of Magnetic Therapy, Los Angeles, January 21–23, 2000).

5.   R. Rogachevsky, "Use of Magnets in Orthopedics: Research on Post-Traumatic Arthritis and Fracture Healing" (paper presented at the sixth annual meeting of the North American Academy of Magnetic Therapy, Los Angeles, January 21–23, 2000).

6.   M. Markov, "Use of EMFs in Anti-Angiogenesis" (paper presented at the sixth annual meeting of the North American Academy of Magnetic Therapy, Los Angeles, January 21–23, 2000).

7.   B. Sisken, "Static Magnets and Nerve Regeneration in Vitro" (paper presented at the fifth annual meeting of the North American Academy of Magnetic Therapy, Los Angeles, January 22–24, 1999), audiotape.

8.   J. I. Jacobson et al., "The Effect of Magnetic Resonance on the Regeneration of the Sciatic Nerve of Mice in Vitro" (paper available from Dr. B. B. Saxena, Cornell University Medical Center, Room A267, 1300 York Ave., New York, NY 10021).

9.   Telephone conversation with Dr. Jerry Jacobson, Jacobson Resonance Enterprises, Boca Raton, Fla., June 17, 1999.

10.   Telephone conversation with Dr. David Stokesbary, Advanced Magnetic Research Institute, Laguna Niguel, Calif., September 9, 1999.

11.   J. Carper, *Miracle Cures* (New York: HarperCollins, 1998), 26.

INDEX

Index

Index

ABOUT THE AUTHOR

Sherry Kahn, M.P.H., is a health educator, writer, and communications consultant, who resides in Santa Monica, California. She received her master's degree in public health from the University of Michigan, is a former UCLA Medical Center principal editor, and is the author of *The Nurse's Meditative Journal* and the coauthor of *Healing Yourself: A Nurse's Guide to Self-Care and Renewal.*

Kahn first became interested in natural pain relief tools while working as a massage therapist. Having spent more than two decades with one foot in mainstream medicine and the other in alternative medicine, she is delighted to see the chasm between the two lessening. She particularly enjoys working on integrative medicine projects—those that combine the best of all medicines.